CRQs for the Final FRCA

CRQs for the Final FRCA

M. Ashraf Akuji
Specialty Registrar in Anaesthesia, North West School of Anaesthesia, UK

Fiona Martin
Specialty Registrar in Anaesthesia, North West School of Anaesthesia, UK

David Chambers
Consultant in Anaesthesia, Salford Royal NHS Foundation Trust, Salford, UK

Elizabeth Thomas
Consultant in Anaesthesia and Intensive Care Medicine, Stockport NHS Foundation Trust, Stockport, UK

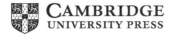
CAMBRIDGE
UNIVERSITY PRESS

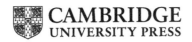

Shaftesbury Road, Cambridge CB2 8EA, United Kingdom

One Liberty Plaza, 20th Floor, New York, NY 10006, USA

477 Williamstown Road, Port Melbourne, VIC 3207, Australia

314–321, 3rd Floor, Plot 3, Splendor Forum, Jasola District Centre, New Delhi – 110025, India

103 Penang Road, #05–06/07, Visioncrest Commercial, Singapore 238467

Cambridge University Press is part of Cambridge University Press & Assessment, a department of the University of Cambridge.

We share the University's mission to contribute to society through the pursuit of education, learning and research at the highest international levels of excellence.

www.cambridge.org
Information on this title: www.cambridge.org/9781108705288

DOI: 10.1017/9781108668958

First published 2019

A catalogue record for this publication is available from the British Library

Library of Congress Cataloging-in-Publication data
Names: Akuji, M. Ashraf, author. | Martin, Fiona (Specialty registrar in anesthesia), author. | Chambers, David, 1979– author. | Thomas, Elizabeth (Consultant in anesthesia), author.
Title: CRQs for the final FRCA / M. Ashraf Akuji, Fiona Martin, David Chambers, Elizabeth Thomas.
Description: Cambridge, United Kingdom ; New York, NY : Cambridge University Press, 2019. | Includes bibliographical references and index.
Identifiers: LCCN 2019000405 | ISBN 9781108705288 (alk. paper)
Subjects: | MESH: Anesthesia | Analgesia | United Kingdom | Examination Question
Classification: LCC RD82.3 | NLM WO 218.2 | DDC 617.9/6076–dc23
LC record available at https://lccn.loc.gov/2019000405

ISBN   978-1-108-70528-8   Paperback

....

MAA: To those who have taught me over the years and given me the opportunity to succeed. To my wife for her support and my children for their smiles, which keep me going.

FM: To my mum, dad and brother for all their support, y a mí esposo Diego por ser mi mejor amigo.

DC: To my parents, Ruth and Chris, for their support and for setting unachievable publication targets.

ET: In memory of my mother, Brenda, and for my husband, Andrew – two people who have always believed in me.

All: We would also like to 'thank' the driver who knocked Dave off his bike, thus enabling the extended period of laptop time that followed, and expedited the publication of this book.

Authors' Note

Many of the questions give the patient a name. None of these are the real name of a patient. The scenarios represent a combination of the authors' experiences of similar cases and the names are those of our colleagues, friends and relatives around the North West region who have been supportive with the production of this book or our anaesthetic training, with our thanks to them.

Contents

Foreword by Sarah Thornton   *page* ix

Introduction		1
Paper 1 **Questions**		3
Paper 2 **Questions**		15
Paper 3 **Questions**		26
Paper 4 **Questions**		38
Paper 5 **Questions**		50
Paper 6 **Questions**		62
Paper 7 **Questions**		75
Paper 8 **Questions**		88
Paper 9 **Questions**		99
Paper 10 **Questions**		111

Paper 1 **Answers**   123
Paper 2 **Answers**   149
Paper 3 **Answers**   178
Paper 4 **Answers**   206
Paper 5 **Answers**   235
Paper 6 **Answers**   263
Paper 7 **Answers**   291
Paper 8 **Answers**   322
Paper 9 **Answers**   350
Paper 10 **Answers**   379

Index   410

Foreword

During my time as an educator in the North West, I have seen the impact of trying to do exams, hold down a difficult and demanding job and find time for family and friends. The Final FRCA written paper is changing in 2019 with the addition of a new type of question: the Constructed Response Question. Post-graduate anaesthesia exams are challenging, and the uncertainty of change only adds to trainees' anxiety.

All four authors are eminently qualified, being the backbone faculty of the North West Final FRCA Exam Practice Course, which boasts results that have been consistently above the national average for both written and structured oral examinations. They have put their considerable experience, and a good deal of time and energy, into providing you with a comprehensive and practical set of 10 sample CRQ papers. Simply laid out, easy to read and with sample answers that are easy to assimilate, it offers the perfect revision guide and is quite simply the best choice to help you through the new style of Final written paper.

Good luck!

Sarah Thornton
Head of the School of Anaesthesia, Health Education North West

Introduction

Prior to 2019, the Royal College of Anaesthetists' (RCoA) Final FRCA written paper consisted of two parts: the combined Multiple-Choice Question (MCQ) and Single Best Answer (SBA) question paper, and the Structured Answer Question (SAQ) paper.

Why Have Two Types of Papers?

The MCQ/SBA paper is a 'selected-response paper', where the candidate is given a selection of answers from which to choose. This form of questioning allows the examiners to sample the curriculum widely and can be computer marked, but there is a risk of candidates scoring simply by guessing.

The SAQ paper is a 'constructed response paper', where candidates have to produce the correct words or phrases to score marks. The theoretical advantage of using this type of questioning is that it allows candidates to demonstrate a complex, in-depth understanding of topics. However, a smaller proportion of the curriculum is tested by the SAQ paper, and candidates' answers are very laborious to mark.

Why Change from the SAQ?

The SAQ paper has been used for over two decades. During this time, it has evolved from an essay question to a question divided into three to four sub-questions. The pressure to dispense with the SAQ has come from the time-consuming nature of the paper marking, at a time when examiners are increasingly difficult to recruit. In 2015, the RCoA announced its intention to replace SAQs with a new format of question, the Constructed Response Question (CRQ). In 2019 the RCoA introduced a hybrid SAQ/CRQ paper; CRQs are to completely replace SAQs by September 2020, with the aim of moving towards computer-based marking thereafter.

What Are CRQs?

The RCoA describes their idea of CRQs as consisting of

- Open-ended short answer questions with precise answer templates;
- Most commonly used to assess knowledge and application-level cognitive skills;
- Can include real-world artefacts (graphs, images, scenarios, cases);
- Typically consist of three to five sub-sections, often including a clinical scenario;
- Sub-sections increase in complexity and difficulty as the question progresses.

In our view, the six pilot CRQs released by the RCoA are a little more structured than their predecessor SAQs. One- or two-word answers to short sentences are required.

What Have We Learnt from Writing This Book?

During the writing of this book, we aimed to 'get into the head' of the RCoA examiner. From what we have learnt, we think we can give you a few tips for the CRQ paper:

- Like the SAQ paper, one to two questions per paper are likely to be difficult, one to two easy and the rest moderate. The pass mark will reflect this, so if you are finding a question particularly hard – don't worry!

- Although it has not been confirmed at the time of writing this book, the most likely format of the CRQ paper is to mirror that of the current SAQ, i.e. one question from each of the mandatory units of training (neuro, cardiac, paediatric, critical care, pain and obstetric), four from general duties and two from optional units. We have reflected this when writing the question papers.
- The easiest way of writing a CRQ question is by basing it on a recent *BJA Education* article or on guidance published by the RCoA, AAGBI or other national bodies. As part of your revision, you should consider reading the last few years' *BJA Education* articles, major clinical guidelines and national audit reports.
- When you are asked to list the clinical features of acromegaly, or the physiological consequences of obesity, answer widely across all body systems. If you give five cardiovascular features, you are unlikely to get all the marks. It is more likely that there will be, for example, 2 marks for cardiovascular, 1 for metabolic, 1 for airway and 1 for gastrointestinal.
- Where a question asks for three clinical features, you are likely only to get marks for the **first three** that you write down – so make those your best ones!
- The easiest way to write a CRQ is to adapt an old SAQ, so make sure you look through the previous SAQ papers published by the RCoA on their website.
- The RCoA have stated their intention to include clinical data (e.g. arterial blood gases) and radiological pictures in their CRQs. In writing this book, we found that anatomy is most easily assessed in a 'label the diagram' type question and suspect that this is a direction that the examiners will also move in.
- Unlike the SAQ, there is plenty of time to complete the CRQ paper. Most importantly, there is time to read the question carefully. So, if the question says the word 'specific', you must answer specifically. There are unlikely to be any marks for woolly answers such as 'ABCDE assessment'.

We hope you find this book a useful revision and examination practice tool!

Paper 1

Question 1.

Anton is a 32-year-old man who was found unconscious and brought to the Emergency Department. His past medical history includes craniopharyngioma (resected as a child) and a ventriculoperitoneal (VP) shunt. The neurosurgeon suspects the patient has hydrocephalus secondary to a blocked VP shunt.

a) List two other possible **neurological** diagnoses based on the information above. (2 marks)

   1. _____

   2. _____

b) List two symptoms and four signs of an acute rise in intracranial pressure (ICP). (6 marks)

   Symptoms:

   1. _____

   2. _____

   Signs:

   1. _____

   2. _____

   3. _____

   4. _____

c) Complete the following table regarding cerebrospinal fluid (CSF) flow. (5 marks)

Table 1.1c **Production and flow of CSF**

1.	Site of CSF production			
2.	Flows to		Through	
3.	Flows to		Through	
4.	Flows to subarachnoid space through		And	
5.	Absorption takes place at			

d) Name three roles of CSF. (3 marks)

   1. _____

   2. _____

   3. _____

e) The neurosurgeon suspects that the VP shunt is infected and removes it. She inserts an external ventricular drain (EVD) to relieve the raised ICP and prescribes a setting of $+15$ cmH$_2$O. How would you set up the collecting burette? (2 marks)

   _____

   _____

f) List two complications associated with EVDs. (2 marks)

1. _____

2. _____

Question 2.

David, a 56-year-old man, is listed for elective repair of a large incisional hernia. He has a background history of dilated cardiomyopathy.

a) Complete the following table (with low, normal or high) describing the pathological features of the three World Health Organization–recognised types of cardiomyopathy. (3 marks)

Table 1.2a **Types of cardiomyopathy**

	Dilated	Hypertrophic	Restrictive
Cardiac output	Low		
Stroke volume		Low	
Contractility			Normal

b) Although most commonly idiopathic, list three other causes of dilated cardiomyopathy. (3 marks)

1. _____

2. _____

3. _____

At the pre-operative clinic, David's symptoms of heart failure appear to be well controlled, and his chest is clear on auscultation. He takes 10 mg of Ramipril daily and last attended cardiology clinic more than 12 months ago.

c) List three investigations you would request prior to listing David for his elective procedure. (3 marks)

1. _____

2. _____

3. _____

Following relevant investigations, David proceeds to surgery.

d) Aside from AAGBI-recommended standard monitoring, what further monitoring and access would you instigate prior to anaesthetising David for his incisional hernia repair? (3 marks)

1. _____

2. _____

3. _____

e) State the principles by which you would manage his **cardiovascular physiology** intra-operatively. (5 marks)

1. _____

2. _____

3. _____

4. _____

5. _____

Your consultant suggests performing an epidural block for David's surgery due to the size of the hernia.

f) List two advantages and one disadvantage of neuraxial blockade **specific to cardiovascular physiology** in dilated cardiomyopathy. (3 marks)

Advantages:

1. _____

2. _____

Disadvantage:

1. _____

Question 3.

Rachel is a 53-year-old woman who has spent 10 days ventilated on the Intensive Care Unit (ICU) for a community-acquired pneumonia. She is weaning from mechanical ventilation, having had a tracheostomy sited. However, you notice she appears weak and struggles to lift her arms.

a) Define ICU-acquired weakness (ICUAW). (1 mark)

_____

b) List the three classes of ICUAW. (3 marks)

1. _____

2. _____

3. _____

c) List six risk factors for the development of ICUAW. (6 marks)

1. _____

2. _____

3. _____

4. _____

5. _____

6. _____

d) List four clinical features of ICUAW. (4 marks)

1. _____

2. _____

3. _____

4. _____

e) List four clinical investigations that aid the diagnosis and differentiation of ICUAW. (4 marks)

1. _____

2. _____

3. _____

4. _____

f) What proportion of patients diagnosed with ICUAW will die during their hospital admission? (1 mark)

g) What proportion of patients who survive their hospital admission will achieve a complete recovery? (1 mark)

Question 4.

You review Frank, a 3-year-old boy on your day-case list who will be undergoing a circumcision. He weighs 15 kg. His parents want to discuss analgesia and have read an information leaflet about caudal analgesia.

a) List four other analgesic options that could be considered in this case. (4 marks)

1. _____
2. _____
3. _____
4. _____

b) Complete the labels (i–vi) on the following figure. (3 marks)

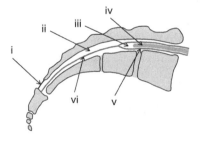

Figure 1.4b Anatomy of the caudal space

   i. _____
  ii. _____
 iii. _____
 iv. _____
  v. _____
 vi. _____

c) Where does the dural sac normally end in a child of this age? (1 mark)

d) List four complications of caudal blockade. (4 marks)

1. _____
2. _____
3. _____
4. _____

e) State the name, concentration and volume of local anaesthetic agent you would use for the caudal in this case, according to the Armitage 'rules'. (3 marks)

Name _____

Concentration _____

Volume _____

f) List two drugs (with doses) that could be added to your local anaesthetic mixture to prolong the duration or quality of the block. (2 marks)

1. _____

2. _____

g) Following surgery, the recovery nurse is concerned that Frank is in pain. List three methods of assessing pain in a child of this age group. (3 marks)

1. _____

2. _____

3. _____

Question 5.

Lorna is a 30-year-old nulliparous woman on the maternity unit. She has been classified as 'high risk' and is on continuous cardiotocography (CTG) monitoring.

a) List three features of the foetal heart rate (FHR) that are used to define and interpret CTG traces. (3 marks)

1. _____

2. _____

3. _____

b) How may a CTG trace be categorised? (3 marks)

1. _____

2. _____

3. _____

Following review of the CTG, the obstetric team decides to take a foetal blood sample (FBS).

c) Complete the following table regarding the classification for FBS results. (6 marks)

Table 1.5c **Classification of FBS results**

	pH	Lactate
Normal		
Borderline		
Abnormal		

The FBS is abnormal, and a decision is made to undertake a caesarean section.

d) According to the National Institute for Health and Care Excellence's categorisation of the urgency of a caesarean section, explain each category below (no marks will be awarded for time to delivery). (4 marks)

Category 1. _____

Category 2. _____

Category 3. _____

Category 4. _____

e) Which women may be offered a planned caesarean section? (4 marks)

1. _____

2. _____

3. _____

4. _____

Question 6.

You are called to the Emergency Department to assess Ian, a 63-year-old man with known chronic obstructive pulmonary disease (COPD). He has sustained fractures to his ninth, tenth and eleventh ribs on his right-hand side following a fall but has no other injuries.

a) List five pulmonary complications that may result following multiple rib fractures. (5 marks)

1. _____

2. _____

3. _____

4. _____

5. _____

b) Other than additional analgesia, list two measures you would instigate to help prevent pulmonary complications in this patient. (2 marks)

1. _____

2. _____

c) Despite regular paracetamol and codeine, Ian remains in pain. State which drugs you would add next to Ian's analgesic regimen. (2 marks)

1. _____

2. _____

Despite all pharmacological attempts to make Ian comfortable, he remains in pain.

d) List three regional anaesthetic techniques that could provide analgesia in this case, and for each technique, give one advantage and one disadvantage. (9 marks)

Table 1.6d **Advantages and disadvantages of regional techniques used in the management of rib fractures**

	Regional anaesthetic technique	Advantage	Disadvantage
1.			
2.			
3.			

e) What are the indications for surgical rib fixation? (2 marks)

Question 7.

Bronagh is an 86-year-old woman admitted for an elective total hip replacement due to osteoarthritis, which you opt to perform under spinal anaesthesia. She has a background history of hypertension. During the procedure, there is a sudden change in her observations associated with cementing of the hip joint.

a) Complete the following table defining grades one and two of bone cement implantation syndrome (BCIS). (6 marks)

Table 1.7a **Grading of BCIS**

BCIS grade	SpO_2 (%)	Systolic blood pressure (% reduction)	Loss of consciousness (yes or no)
1			
2			

b) List the defining feature of grade 3 BCIS. (1 mark)

c) Aside from systemic hypertension, list three further **patient** risk factors for the development of BCIS. (3 marks)

1. _____

2. _____

3. _____

d) Although the exact causative mechanism is poorly understood, summarise the pathophysiological mechanism through which **hypoxia** (2 marks) and **cardiovascular collapse** (2 marks) are thought to occur.

e) During cementing, Bronagh becomes hypoxic and hypotensive. You have called for help. Describe your immediate management. (4 marks)

f) Aside from not using cement, list two surgical techniques that can be employed to reduce the risk of BCIS. (2 marks)

1. _____

2. _____

Question 8.

Louise, a 32-year-old woman, is referred to an endocrinologist with symptoms of hyperthyroidism.

a) What are the four steps involved in synthesis of thyroid hormones? (4 marks)

1. _____

2. _____

3. _____

4. _____

b) List six symptoms of hyperthyroidism. (6 marks)

1. _____

2. _____

3. _____

4. _____

5. _____

6. _____

c) List two causes of hyperthyroidism. (2 marks)

1. _____

2. _____

d) What would you expect her thyroid function tests to show? (2 marks)

_____

_____

The patient has biochemically confirmed hyperthyroidism. She is rendered euthyroid pharmacologically.

e) List two drugs which she may have been given. (2 marks)

1. _____

2. _____

Three months later, Louise is referred for a surgical thyroidectomy and attends pre-operative assessment clinic. Louise is concerned about the risk of surgical complications following her thyroidectomy.

f) List four serious post-operative complications specific to thyroidectomy. (4 marks)

1. _____

2. _____

3. _____

4. _____

Question 9.

You are asked to review Dawn, a 56-year-old woman, in pre-operative clinic. She is awaiting a laparoscopic hemicolectomy for cancer. In the referral letter, her general practitioner notes that she is anaemic.

a) List four causes of chronic anaemia. (4 marks)

1. _____
2. _____
3. _____
4. _____

She has the following blood results: Hb 76 g/L, mean cell volume (MCV) 72 fL (normal range 77–95 fL), serum ferritin 8 µg/L (normal range 15–300 µg/L).

b) Interpret the blood results. (1 mark)

_____

c) List four clinical features of severe anaemia that you might find from the history and examination. (4 marks)

1. _____
2. _____
3. _____
4. _____

d) The proposed date of surgery is 4 weeks away. What would you prescribe to improve her anaemia? (1 mark)

_____

The patient arrives on the day of surgery. Blood tests taken the previous day reveal an improvement in her anaemia: Hb 92 g/L.

e) List eight measures that could be taken in the perioperative period to reduce her risk of requiring an allogenic transfusion. (8 marks)

1. _____
2. _____
3. _____
4. _____
5. _____
6. _____
7. _____
8. _____

f) List two risks of allogenic transfusion **specific** to cancer surgery. (2 marks)

1. _____
2. _____

Question 10.

Laura is a 75-year-old woman who is due to undergo electroconvulsive therapy (ECT) for severe depression.

a) For each psychoactive drug that the patient is taking, as listed in the table below, state the drug class (in full) and a drug interaction of relevance to anaesthetists. (6 marks)

Table 1.10a **Antidepressant drugs**

Drug	Drug class	Drug interaction
Fluoxetine		
Amitriptyline		
Phenelzine		

b) Name the two positions in which ECT electrodes may be applied to the scalp. What are the advantages of each position? (4 marks)

Position: _____

Advantage: _____

Position: _____

Advantage: _____

c) Describe the cardiovascular response of the autonomic nervous system to ECT. (4 marks)

_____

_____

_____

_____

d) Name four relative contraindications to ECT. (4 marks)

1. _____

2. _____

3. _____

4. _____

e) Name two methods used to prevent physical injury to the patient during ECT. (2 marks)

1. _____

2. _____

Question 11.

You are called from a neighbouring theatre to assist a colleague who suspects that his patient, Natalie, has suffered an anaphylactic reaction.

a) List four clinical features that would lead the anaesthetist to suspect anaphylaxis. (4 marks)

1. _____

2. _____

3. _____

4. _____

b) List the **classes** of the four most common triggers for perioperative anaphylaxis. (4 marks)

1. _____

2. _____

3. _____

4. _____

c) What is the incidence of perioperative anaphylaxis in the United Kingdom? (1 mark)

_____

d) Describe your initial clinical and pharmacological management (including doses) of this situation. (4 marks)

_____

_____

_____

_____

e) Regarding immunology, what type of hypersensitivity reaction is anaphylaxis? (1 mark) Describe the underlying immunological process. (4 marks)

Hypersensitivity reaction:_____

Immunological process:_____

_____

_____

The patient is stabilised and transferred to the critical care unit. Blood tests have been taken in preparation for referral to the allergy service.

f) What test was taken, and what are the recommended timings for this blood test? (2 marks)

_____

_____

Question 12.

Maurice, a 78-year-old man, is listed for an elective repair of a 6 cm infrarenal abdominal aortic aneurysm (AAA). His past medical history includes chronic obstructive pulmonary disease, mitral stenosis, hypertension and a biventricular pacemaker with defibrillator (cardiac resynchronisation device, CRD).

a) List six advantages of an endovascular aneurysm repair (EVAR) compared to an open repair for this patient. (6 marks)

1. _____

2. _____

3. _____

4. _____

5. _____

6. _____

b) List four risk factors for acute kidney injury (AKI) for patients undergoing any EVAR procedure. (4 marks)

1. _____

2. _____

3. _____

4. _____

c) List four perioperative measures to prevent AKI following EVAR. (4 marks)

1. _____

2. _____

3. _____

4. _____

d) What are the indications for implanting a CRD? (2 marks) List four perioperative implications of this device. (4 marks)

Indications for CRD:

1. _____

2. _____

Perioperative implications:

1. _____

2. _____

3. _____

4. _____

Paper 2

Question 1.

Julian, a 43-year-old roofer, has fallen from the roof of a two-storey building. He sustains a series of cervical spinal fractures. An anterior–posterior cervical fixation is planned with intra-operative spinal cord monitoring.

a) Name the two types of spinal cord monitoring. (2 marks)

1. _____
2. _____

b) List two anaesthetic consequences specific to cases involving intra-operative spinal cord monitoring. (2 marks)

1. _____
2. _____

c) List four options for body support of the patient when in the prone position. (4 marks)

1. _____
2. _____
3. _____
4. _____

d) List four neurological complications of the prone position. (4 marks)

1. _____
2. _____
3. _____
4. _____

e) Inadequate prone positioning may lead to abdominal compression. List six non-neurological complications of abdominal compression in the prone position. (6 marks)

1. _____
2. _____
3. _____
4. _____
5. _____
6. _____

f) During the case, whilst in the prone position, Julian is accidentally extubated. What would first alert you to this problem, and how would you initially manage the airway? (2 marks)

_____

_____

Question 2.

Lawrence, a 56-year-old man, is listed for an elective laparoscopic cholecystectomy for gallstone disease. He received an orthotopic heart transplant 12 years previously.

a) List four physiological perioperative implications of a denervated heart. (4 marks)

   1. _____
   2. _____
   3. _____
   4. _____

b) List four pharmacological perioperative implications of a denervated heart. (4 marks)

   1. _____
   2. _____
   3. _____
   4. _____

c) List two pre-operative investigations that you would request for this patient. (2 marks)

   1. _____
   2. _____

d) List the anaesthetic considerations specific to the previous cardiac transplant. (4 marks)

   1. _____
   2. _____
   3. _____
   4. _____

e) Lawrence currently takes tacrolimus and mycophenolate mofetil. How will you manage the patient's immunosuppression in the perioperative period? (3 marks)

   _____
   _____
   _____

f) List three long-term health issues that may occur as a result of receiving a cardiac transplant. (3 marks)

   1. _____
   2. _____
   3. _____

Question 3.

a) Which body is responsible for regulating and overseeing organ donation in the UK? (1 mark)

   _____

b) What is the UK definition of death? (1 mark)

   _____

c) List the four preconditions that need to be met prior to brainstem death testing. (4 marks)

   1. _____
   2. _____
   3. _____
   4. _____

d) At what stage during the brainstem testing process is the legal time of death? (1 mark)

_____

e) List four common physiological derangements that may occur following brainstem death in individuals awaiting organ donation. (4 marks) For each, explain the patho-physiological cause. (4 marks)

Physiological derangement 1: _____

Pathophysiological cause 1: _____

Physiological derangement 2: _____

Pathophysiological cause 2: _____

Physiological derangement 3: _____

Pathophysiological cause 3: _____

Physiological derangement 4: _____

Pathophysiological cause 4: _____

f) Describe the normal physiological response to hypercapnoea ($P_aCO_2 > 6.0$ kPa). (4 marks)

_____

_____

_____

_____

Prior to performing the apnoea test, an arterial blood gas confirms a P_aCO_2 of 6.0 kPa.

g) What is the minimum increase in P_aCO_2 required to confirm a positive apnoea test? (1 mark)

_____

Question 4.

Andrew, a 9-month-old boy, is brought by paramedics to the Emergency Department. You are asked to assess him as he is lethargic and is only responsive to painful stimuli. His mother is in attendance and is reluctant to allow nursing staff to undress the child. On examination, there are several bruises on the child's arms and legs of differing ages. You suspect non-accidental injury (NAI).

a) List the four categories of child abuse. (4 marks)

1. _____

2. _____

3. _____

4. _____

b) List six risk factors for child abuse. (6 marks)

1. _____

2. _____

3. _____

4. _____

5. _____

6. _____

c) Aside from NAI, what is your differential diagnosis of this patient's clinical presentation? (6 marks)

1. _____
2. _____
3. _____
4. _____
5. _____
6. _____

d) With whom should you discuss your child safeguarding concerns? (1 mark)

_____

e) State the type of staff that should be undertaking each of the following levels of child protection training, and for each, give an example of a member of **theatre staff**. (3 marks)

Level 1. _____
Example: _____
Level 2. _____
Example: _____
Level 3. _____
Example: _____

Question 5.

Dani is a 32-year-old woman who is 26 weeks pregnant and is found to have a blood pressure (BP) of 160/104 mmHg in antenatal clinic. Her booking BP was 122/74 mmHg. Her urine dipstick is negative for protein, and she is diagnosed with gestational hypertension.

a) List four diagnostic criteria for gestational hypertension. (4 marks)

1. _____
2. _____
3. _____
4. _____

Dani is admitted to the ward for BP control and commenced on oral labetalol. A history of hypertension in a previous pregnancy means she is at high risk of pre-eclampsia, and she is commenced on aspirin.

b) State three other medical conditions which increase a woman's risk of developing pre-eclampsia. (3 marks)

1. _____
2. _____
3. _____

Dani's BP is managed with oral labetalol and preparations are made to discharge her home. She is advised to seek immediate advice if she experiences symptoms of pre-eclampsia.

c) List four common **symptoms** of pre-eclampsia. (4 marks)

1. _____
2. _____
3. _____
4. _____

On a subsequent admission, Dani is found to have a BP of 157/110 mmHg with significant proteinuria, and a diagnosis of pre-eclampsia is made.

d) What is the definition of significant proteinuria? (1 mark)

_____

e) List three biochemical or haematological abnormalities that may be found in patients with severe pre-eclampsia. (3 marks)

1. _____
2. _____
3. _____

f) Oral labetalol fails to control her BP adequately. Name two parenteral drugs **with doses** which are used primarily to control blood pressure in severe pre-eclampsia. (2 marks)

1. _____
2. _____

Dani continues to deteriorate despite medical management. Preparations are being made to deliver the foetus when Dani suddenly loses consciousness and has a tonic-clonic seizure.

g) State the drug that should be given, including the initial dose, maintenance dose and duration. (3 marks)

Drug: _____

Initial dose: _____

Maintenance dose/duration: _____

Question 6.

Jane, a 34-year-old woman, is referred to pain clinic by her general practitioner with suspected trigeminal neuralgia.

a) List three symptoms and signs commonly associated with trigeminal neuralgia. (3 marks)

1. _____
2. _____
3. _____

b) List four other medical conditions which may be considered in the differential diagnosis of unilateral facial pain. (4 marks)

1. _____
2. _____
3. _____
4. _____

c) The patient undergoes a magnetic resonance (MR) scan of her brain which demonstrates demyelination of the trigeminal nerve. List the three most likely causes of this MR abnormality. (3 marks)

1. _____
2. _____
3. _____

The patient's GP initially tried to manage the trigeminal neuralgia pharmacologically.

d) What is the first-line agent used in the treatment of trigeminal neuralgia? (1 mark)

_____

Pharmacological management failed to control Jane's symptoms. Given the abnormality on the MR scan, she is referred to a neurosurgeon.

e) List the three surgical options available, and give an advantage and disadvantage for each. (9 marks)

Table 2.6e **Surgical options for the management of trigeminal neuralgia**

	Surgical option	Advantage	Disadvantage
1.			
2.			
3.			

Question 7.

You are asked to anaesthetise Victoria, a 65-year-old woman with long-standing rheumatoid arthritis, for a total knee replacement. She takes prednisolone 15 mg daily.

a) Other than the knee joint, list two joints which are commonly affected in rheumatoid arthritis. (2 marks)

1. _____

2. _____

b) List three reasons why patients with rheumatoid arthritis may have a difficult airway. (3 marks)

1. _____

2. _____

3. _____

c) List the extra-articular features of rheumatoid arthritis, and for each feature, state the anaesthetic relevance. (10 marks)

Table 2.7c **Extra-articular features of rheumatoid arthritis**

	Extra–articular feature	Anaesthetic relevance
1.		
2.		
3.		
4.		
5.		
6.		
7.		
8.		
9.		
10.		

d) List three clinical features and corresponding perioperative consequences of long-term corticosteroid therapy. (3 marks)

1. _____

2. _____

3. _____

e) List two biological disease-modifying drugs used in the treatment of rheumatoid arthritis. (2 marks)

1. _____

2. _____

Question 8.

Adam is a 10-year-old boy who presents to the Emergency Department with abdominal pain. He is subsequently listed by the general surgeons for an emergency appendicectomy. His father has malignant hyperthermia (MH), and Adam has never been tested. The father is concerned that Adam may have inherited the disease.

a) What is the Mendelian inheritance of MH? (1 mark)

_____

b) List the two known triggers of MH. (2 marks)

1. _____

2. _____

c) Name a disease associated with MH. (1 mark)

_____

d) Outline how a lower motor neuron action potential normally results in muscle contraction. (6 marks)

_____

_____

_____

_____

_____

_____

e) What is the abnormality in MH, and what effect does this abnormality have? (2 marks)

_____

_____

f) List four clinical features of MH. (4 marks)

1. _____

2. _____

3. _____

4. _____

Due to the emergency nature of the surgery, there is insufficient time to test Adam for MH.

g) List two measures you would take to prepare your anaesthetic machine in advance of anaesthetising a patient with MH. (2 marks)

1. _____

2. _____

h) The child's father wishes to know how his other children could be tested for MH. What are the two options? (2 marks)

1. _____

2. _____

Question 9.

Ben, a 30-year-old intravenous drug user, is listed for an incision and drainage of a groin abscess. He is known to have human immunodeficiency virus (HIV). Whilst siting the cannula, you suffer a needlestick injury.

a) State the risk of developing hepatitis B, hepatitis C and HIV following exposure to infected blood via a needlestick injury. (3 marks)

Hepatitis B _____

Hepatitis C _____

HIV _____

b) List four features which increase the risk of HIV transmission from a needlestick injury. (4 marks)

1. _____

2. _____

3. _____

4. _____

c) What should your immediate actions be following the needlestick injury? (2 marks)

_____

d) What specific treatments are available to you following a needlestick injury to protect against hepatitis B, hepatitis C and HIV? (3 marks)

Hepatitis B: _____

Hepatitis C: _____

HIV: _____

e) When should the treatment for HIV exposure be started (1 mark), and how long is the course? (1 mark)

_____

f) The most recent UK guidelines recommend using a combination drug following HIV exposure. State the name of this drug, and give either the name or class of the two constituent drugs. (3 marks)

_____

_____

_____

g) Give three common side effects of these drugs. (3 marks)

_____

_____

_____

Question 10.

Susannah, a 20-year-old woman, is admitted for elective laparoscopic treatment of endometriosis. On pre-operative assessment, she informs you that she has previously suffered with post-operative nausea and vomiting (PONV).

a) What is the accepted time frame for a diagnosis of post-operative nausea and vomiting? (1 mark)

_____

b) List four patient-related potential complications of PONV. (4 marks)

1. _____
2. _____
3. _____
4. _____

c) List the factors that make up the simplified Apfel score. (4 marks)

1. _____
2. _____
3. _____
4. _____

d) Susannah's calculated Apfel score is 3. What is her percentage risk of developing PONV? (1 mark)

_____

e) Complete the following table regarding five drugs that may be used in the management of PONV. (10 marks)

Table 2.10e **Drugs used in the management of PONV**

Drug name	Dose	Receptor activity in PONV	Timing of dose (pre-induction/ induction/end of surgery)
Ondansetron	4 mg		
Droperidol			
Dexamethasone		Unknown	
Aprepitant	40 mg		
Metoclopramide		Dopamine D_2 antagonist	Induction

Question 11.

Tom, a 35-year-old man, is to receive total intravenous anaesthesia (TIVA).

a) List six indications for TIVA. (6 marks)

1. _____
2. _____
3. _____

4. _____

5. _____

6. _____

b) State the two pharmacokinetic models most commonly used for propofol. (2 marks)

1. _____

2. _____

c) Regarding pharmacokinetics, outline the three-compartment model. State the compartment into which intravenous drug is administered and the compartment from which the drug is eliminated. (5 marks)

_____

_____

_____

_____

_____

d) List five safety features of a Target Controlled Infusion (TCI) pump. (5 marks)

1. _____

2. _____

3. _____

4. _____

5. _____

e) Define the term *zero-order kinetics*. Give an example of a drug that follows zero-order kinetics. (2 marks)

Zero-order kinetics: _____

Drug example: _____

Question 12.

You are asked to anaesthetise Michael, a 14-year-old boy who sustained a pellet injury to his eye an hour ago. The surgeons would like to operate straightaway to save his vision.

a) Complete the labels (i–viii) on the following figure. (4 marks)

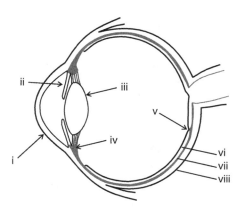

Figure 2.12a Anatomy of the eye

i. _____

ii. _____

iii. _____

iv. _____

v. _____

vi. _____

vii. _____

viii. _____

b) Outline the pathway of aqueous humour, from its site of production to the site of absorption. (4 marks)

_____

_____

_____

_____

_____

The child is not adequately fasted, but given the sight-saving nature of the surgery, you decide to proceed using a rapid sequence induction.

c) Which agents that may be used for rapid sequence induction risk increasing intraocular pressure (IOP)? (2 marks)

1. _____

2. _____

d) Name two drugs which attenuate the sympathetic response to laryngoscopy, and give the typical doses needed to achieve this effect. (2 marks)

1. _____

2. _____

e) The surgeon tells you that the IOP is increasing intra-operatively. List four strategies to reduce IOP. (4 marks)

1. _____

2. _____

3. _____

4. _____

f) The globe is now repaired, but the surgeon is concerned about you precipitating an acute rise in IOP when waking the patient. List four strategies for avoiding an acute rise in IOP during emergence and in the post-operative period. (4 marks)

1. _____

2. _____

3. _____

4. _____

Paper 3

Question 1.

Russell, a 32-year-old man, has fallen from his mountain bike at speed. He landed on his head but was wearing a cycle helmet. You are part of the receiving trauma team in the Emergency Department.

a) Russell tells you he cannot move his arms or legs. You proceed to examine Russell, starting with his upper limbs. Complete the table of upper limb myotomes. (4 marks)

Table 3.1a **Myotomes of the upper limb**

Joint/action	Myotome (spinal nerve most strongly associated with movement)
1. Shoulder abduction	
2. Elbow flexion	
3. Elbow extension	
4. Finger adduction	

b) The patient's observations are as follows: heart rate 40 beats/min, blood pressure 80/38 mmHg. Explain these two findings. (2 marks)

1. _____
2. _____

c) Based on the neurological examination, the patient is thought to have a cervical spinal cord injury. List four indications for intubation in this clinical situation. (4 marks)

1. _____
2. _____
3. _____
4. _____

d) List two precautions you would take when **intubating** this patient. (2 marks)

1. _____
2. _____

e) The patient is now intubated and sedated, and you transfer the patient to the critical care unit. List eight aspects of acute critical care management that you would instigate. (8 marks)

1. _____
2. _____
3. _____
4. _____

5. _____

6. _____

7. _____

8. _____

Question 2.

Insiya is a 74-year-old woman who is listed for an emergency laparotomy due to a perforated diverticulum. She has a background history of ischaemic heart disease and is currently on the waiting list for coronary artery bypass grafting. The operation is taking place in a hospital with tertiary cardiac services.

a) Apart from a history of coronary artery disease, which five other features make up Lee's Revised Cardiac Index? (5 marks)

1. _____

2. _____

3. _____

4. _____

5. _____

b) Based on the history provided above, what is the percentage risk of perioperative cardiac complications? (1 mark)

_____

c) The essential requirement for general anaesthesia in ischaemic heart disease is balancing myocardial oxygen supply with myocardial oxygen demand. In the table below, give three factors affecting myocardial oxygen supply and three factors affecting myocardial oxygen demand. (6 marks)

Table 3.2c Factors affecting myocardial oxygen supply and demand

Myocardial oxygen supply	Myocardial oxygen demand

Intra-operatively, Insiya develops ST depression on the five lead ECG. You immediately inform the surgeon. Despite ensuring that there is adequate oxygenation and correcting haemodynamic disturbance, the ECG changes persist. Insiya has a central line in situ and you decide to commence glyceryl trinitrate (GTN).

d) What is the specific pharmacodynamic rationale behind the use of GTN in ischaemic heart disease, and at what dose (µg/min) would you run the infusion? (2 marks)

_____

_____

e) Insiya's lactate continues to increase and her urine output is decreasing. She is hypotensive despite adequate filling. What is the likely diagnosis? (1 mark)

_____

f) Following discussion with your supervising consultant, you decide to commence enoximone. State the drug class and its mechanism of action. (2 marks)

Drug class:_____

Mechanism of action:_____

g) What non-pharmacological treatment options could be considered? (3 marks)

_____

_____

_____

Question 3.

Lauren is a 22-year-old woman who has been sedated and ventilated on the Intensive Care Unit for 4 days following a major trauma. She has been sedated with high-dose propofol and alfentanil. The nurses are concerned that she is showing signs of propofol-related infusion syndrome (PRIS).

a) List seven clinical manifestations of PRIS. (7 marks)

1. _____

2. _____

3. _____

4. _____

5. _____

6. _____

7. _____

b) What is the maximum dose of propofol (mg/kg/h) that should be used as an infusion? (1 mark)

_____

c) In addition to a high-dose propofol infusion, list four risk factors for developing PRIS. (4 marks)

1. _____

2. _____

3. _____

4. _____

d) What specific laboratory findings might be expected in a case of PRIS? (3 marks)

1. _____

2. _____

3. _____

e) List four aspects of your clinical management of this case. (4 marks)

1. _____

2. _____

3. _____

4. _____

f) What is the mortality from PRIS? (1 mark)

_____

Question 4.

A 5-year-old boy, Sebastian, is listed for a bilateral myringotomy and grommet insertion under general anaesthesia. He has Down's syndrome.

a) State the most common genetic abnormality causing Down's syndrome. (1 mark)

_____

b) How is Down's syndrome diagnosed? (2 marks)

1. _____
2. _____

c) List six features of this child's physical appearance that are characteristic of Down's syndrome. (6 marks)

1. _____
2. _____
3. _____
4. _____
5. _____
6. _____

d) Sebastian is known to have had surgery during the first year of life. List four congenital abnormalities associated with Down's syndrome which may have led to surgery. (4 marks)

1. _____
2. _____
3. _____
4. _____

e) Which haematological malignancy are children with Down's syndrome particularly susceptible to? (1 mark)

_____

f) List two common spinal abnormalities found in Down's syndrome. (2 marks)

1. _____
2. _____

g) On examination, Sebastian is thought to have a difficult airway. List four features specific to Down's syndrome which may make airway management more difficult. (4 marks)

1. _____
2. _____
3. _____
4. _____

Question 5.

You are called urgently to the delivery suite to assist in the management of Cindy, a 31-year-old woman who has collapsed during the second stage of labour. You are told that the working diagnosis is amniotic fluid embolism (AFE).

a) List three further **obstetric** and **non-obstetric** causes of maternal collapse in labour. (6 marks)

Obstetric:

1. _____
2. _____
3. _____

Non-obstetric:

1. _____
2. _____
3. _____

b) In the absence of any other clear cause for the collapse, list five clinical features that may aid the diagnosis of AFE according to the United Kingdom Obstetric Surveillance System (UKOSS) criteria. (5 marks)

1. _____
2. _____
3. _____
4. _____
5. _____

c) State the two main theories hypothesised in the mechanism of AFE. (2 marks)

1. _____
2. _____

d) A biphasic response to AFE is commonly described. What are the two key features of the **phase 2** response? (2 marks)

1. _____
2. _____

e) On your arrival, you note that Cindy is unresponsive with no signs of life. List the key points of the immediate management of this patient. (5 marks)

1. _____
2. _____
3. _____
4. _____
5. _____

Question 6.

You are asked to review Sally, a 42-year-old woman, in pain clinic. She has a history of intractable low back pain.

a) Complete the labels (i–vi) on the following figure. (3 marks)

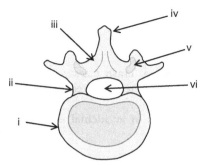

Figure 3.6a Anatomy of the vertebra

i. _____

ii. _____

iii. _____

iv. _____

v. _____

vi. _____

b) List five features in the history and five clinical signs that would suggest serious spinal pathology. (10 marks)

History:

1. _____

2. _____

3. _____

4. _____

5. _____

Clinical signs:

1. _____

2. _____

3. _____

4. _____

5. _____

c) The patient does not have any features of serious spinal pathology, nor does she have lower limb neuropathy. Give three aetiological origins of mechanical back pain. (3 marks)

1. _____

2. _____

3. _____

During the consultation, you recognise that psychosocial factors are making a significant contribution to the patient's pain behaviours.

d) List four psychosocial factors that have been shown to indicate long-term chronicity and disability. (4 marks)

1. _____

2. _____

3. _____

4. _____

Question 7.

Sophie, a 23-year-old woman, has a 'crash Caesarean section' for cord prolapse. You perform an uneventful general anaesthetic. Three hours later, you are asked to review Sophie, as she says she 'was not asleep'.

a) State and define the two classes of accidental awareness under general anaesthesia (AAGA). (4 marks)

Class:_____

Definition:_____

Class:_____

Definition:_____

b) List six factors associated with an increased likelihood of AAGA. (6 marks)

1. _____

2. _____

3. _____

4. _____

5. _____

6. _____

c) How will you manage this clinical situation? (3 marks)

_____

_____

_____

d) List four methods that can be used to monitor depth of anaesthesia. (4 marks)

1. _____

2. _____

3. _____

4. _____

e) Regarding the depth of anaesthesia, state electroencephalogram (EEG) wave patterns consistent with wakefulness, surgical anaesthesia and excessive anaesthesia. (3 marks)

Wakefulness:_____

Surgical anaesthesia:_____

Excessive anaesthesia:_____

Question 8.

On a recent visit to his general practitioner, Glyn, a 58-year-old man, was noted to have unilateral tonsillar hypertrophy. He has been listed for a panendoscopy and biopsy. Your supervising consultant anaesthetist plans to use high-flow nasal oxygen therapy (HFNOT) to facilitate 'tubeless surgery'.

a) List four risk factors for developing oropharyngeal cancer. (4 marks)

1. _____

2. _____

3. _____

4. _____

b) Other than HFNOT, list two strategies to maintain oxygenation during an upper airway panendoscopy. (2 marks)

1. _____

2. _____

c) How will you maintain anaesthesia during this case? (1 mark)

_____

d) Regarding gas delivery, list two differences between HFNOT and conventional nasal cannulae. (2 marks)

1. _____

2. _____

e) State two other perioperative uses of HFNOT. (2 marks)

1. _____

2. _____

f) List five physiological benefits of HFNOT. (5 marks)

1. _____

2. _____

3. _____

4. _____

5. _____

g) List four contraindications to the use of HFNOT. (4 marks)

1. _____

2. _____

3. _____

4. _____

Question 9.

Fiona, a 32-year-old woman, is listed for a laparoscopic right adrenalectomy. An adrenal mass was found when she was investigated for hypertension, and there is a known family history of adrenal tumours.

a) What is the most likely diagnosis? (1 mark)

_____

b) List four substances that this type of adenoma commonly produces. (4 marks)

1. _____

2. _____

3. _____

4. _____

c) List four symptoms that Fiona may experience with this adenoma type. (4 marks)

1. _____

2. _____

3. _____

4. _____

d) During the diagnostic work-up, a blood sample was taken to measure the concentration of a particular substance. What is this substance? (1 mark)

_____

e) List four **specific** measures that you will take to prepare Fiona for surgery. (4 marks)

1. _____

2. _____

3. _____

4. _____

f) Intra-operatively, following surgical handling of the adenoma, the patient becomes hypertensive. List four pharmacological options to manage this. (4 marks)

1. _____

2. _____

3. _____

4. _____

g) Name two health conditions which are associated with developing this type of adenoma. (2 marks)

1. _____

2. _____

Question 10.

Jennifer is a 34-year-old woman who has been admitted with a dental abscess. She has no other past medical history of note, but on pre-operative examination, it is apparent that she cannot open her mouth more than 1 cm due to trismus. You have opted to perform an awake fibre-optic intubation (AFOI).

a) What is the definition of a difficult airway? (1 mark)

_____

b) Aside from patient refusal, list four contraindications to AFOI. (4 marks)

1. _____

2. _____

3. _____

4. _____

c) Complete the following table regarding laryngeal anatomy. (4 marks)

Table 3.10c **Muscles of the larynx**

Muscle(s)	Action
	Tenses vocal cords
Thyroarytenoid and vocalis	
Lateral cricoarytenoid and transverse arytenoid	
	Abduction of vocal cords

d) State the two nerves which innervate the muscles of the vocal cords. (2 marks)

1. _____

2. _____

You have carefully consented Jennifer for an AFOI. Prior to commencing the procedure, you wish to calculate the maximum topical lignocaine dose that you can give.

e) For AFOI, what is the maximum accepted dose of lignocaine (mg/kg)? (1 mark)

_____

f) What percentage of nebulised lignocaine is thought to be systemically absorbed during AFOI? (1 mark)

_____

You have topically anaesthetised Jennifer's supraglottic airway and have opted to perform a trans-tracheal block for subglottic topicalisation.

g) Provide a brief description of how a trans-tracheal block is performed. (3 marks)

_____
_____
_____

The surgery proceeds uneventfully. In accordance with Difficult Airway Society guidelines, you have optimised the patient for extubation.

h) List four other preparations that you would make to ensure a safe extubation. (4 marks)

1. _____

2. _____

3. _____

4. _____

Question 11.

Bashir, a 76-year-old man, is admitted following an episode of colicky abdominal pain. Following investigation, the general surgeons suspect he has an obstructing sigmoid carcinoma and he is listed for a laparotomy. The patient has a history of dementia.

a) List two common causes of dementia in the United Kingdom. (2 marks)

1. _____

2. _____

b) The surgeons have deemed the patient to lack capacity. List the four functional components which must be met for a patient to be deemed to have the capacity to make a decision. (4 marks)

1. _____

2. _____

3. _____

4. _____

c) According to the Mental Capacity Act 2005, if a patient lacks capacity and is unable to consent to a procedure, treatment is carried out in the patient's best interests. List four aspects that should be considered when deciding what is in the patient's best interests. (4 marks)

1. _____
2. _____
3. _____
4. _____

d) With regard to future decision-making about health issues, list two legal options which the patient may have taken prior to the onset of dementia. (2 marks)

1. _____
2. _____

The laparotomy proceeds uneventfully, and the patient is admitted to the critical care unit post-operatively. Over the next 24 hours, his behaviour changes from 'pleasantly confused' to a fluctuating state of worsening confusion, aggression and inattention.

e) Name the diagnosis (1 mark), and list four risk factors for developing this diagnosis. (4 marks)

Diagnosis: _____

Risk factors:

1. _____
2. _____
3. _____
4. _____

f) The patient's behaviour becomes sufficiently challenging to require pharmacological and physical restraint. List two factors that should be considered with regard to a Deprivation of Liberties Safeguarding application. (2 marks)

1. _____
2. _____

g) The patient develops a bronchopneumonia and does not respond to initial antibiotic treatment. A 'not for cardiopulmonary resuscitation' decision is being considered. No relatives or close friends have been identified – which other person should you involve in this decision? (1 mark)

Question 12.

Ruth, a 54-year-old woman, is listed for a deep inferior epigastric perforator (DIEP) free flap breast reconstruction. She has no past medical history other than a mastectomy 6 months previously.

a) State the equation and factors that determine laminar flow of a Newtonian fluid. (3 marks)

_____
_____
_____

b) State three factors which affect blood viscosity, making it a non-Newtonian fluid. (3 mark)

1. _____
2. _____
3. _____

c) List four intra-operative strategies to promote free flap perfusion through vasodilation. (4 marks)

1. _____
2. _____
3. _____
4. _____

d) List two surgical and two non-surgical causes of free flap failure. (4 marks)

Surgical:

1. _____
2. _____

Non-surgical:

1. _____
2. _____

e) The surgical operation note requests 'clinical flap observations'. List six clinical methods for assessing the perfusion of the flap. (6 marks)

1. _____
2. _____
3. _____
4. _____
5. _____
6. _____

Paper 4

Question 1.

Anita, a 30-year-old woman, collapses at work following the onset of a severe headache. On arrival at the Emergency Department, she is confused, and her Glasgow Coma Score is 14 (E4V4M6). A CT brain scan is performed, which shows intraventricular blood. A diagnosis of subarachnoid haemorrhage is made.

a) List the three most common causes of blood in the subarachnoid space. (3 marks)

1. _____
2. _____
3. _____

b) List four risk factors associated with the development of aneurysmal subarachnoid haemorrhage. (4 marks)

1. _____
2. _____
3. _____
4. _____

c) Complete the labels (i–vi) on the following figure. (3 marks)

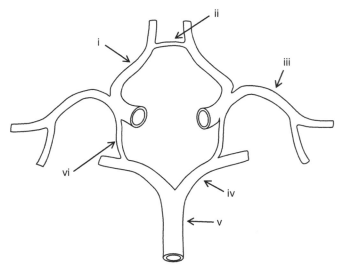

Figure 4.1c Circle of Willis

   i. _____
  ii. _____
 iii. _____

   iv. _____

   v. _____

   vi. _____

d) At which three arteries are berry aneurysms most likely to occur? (3 marks)

   1. _____

   2. _____

   3. _____

e) List the three most common scoring systems in the United Kingdom for grading the severity of aneurysmal subarachnoid haemorrhage. (3 marks)

   1. _____

   2. _____

   3. _____

f) State two early and two late neurological complications of subarachnoid haemorrhage. (4 marks)

Early:

   1. _____

   2. _____

Late:

   1. _____

   2. _____

Question 2.

Steven is a 2-day-old boy who has presented to the Emergency Department following a sudden collapse. He was born by normal vaginal delivery at 37 weeks without complication.

a) A common cause of sudden collapse in a neonate is congenital heart disease. State two other common causes. (2 marks)

   1. _____

   2. _____

b) List four clinical signs that are supportive of a diagnosis of congenital heart disease. (4 marks)

   1. _____

   2. _____

   3. _____

   4. _____

Steven's mother describes a history of irritability and cyanotic spells when feeding and crying. Following examination, you suspect a diagnosis of tetralogy of Fallot.

c) List the tetrad of features seen in this condition. (4 marks)

   1. _____

   2. _____

   3. _____

   4. _____

d) List two conditions associated with tetralogy of Fallot. (2 marks)

1. _____

2. _____

e) Other than feeding, list two other precipitants of a cyanotic episode (tet spell). (2 marks)

1. _____

2. _____

f) Describe the physiological changes in cardiac blood flow that arise during a tet spell. (4 marks)

_____

_____

_____

_____

g) List two ways of managing these cyanotic episodes in the period leading up to corrective surgery. (2 marks)

1. _____

2. _____

Question 3.

You are asked to review Sangeeta in the Emergency Department, a 19-year-old woman with a history of insulin-dependent diabetes. She was found collapsed at home and was previously seen 48 hours ago. Her capillary blood glucose is 21.4 mmol/L.

a) In the space below, list the criteria (in mmol/L) required for a diagnosis of diabetic ketoacidosis (DKA). (3 marks)

Blood glucose greater than:_____

Ketonaemia greater than:_____

Bicarbonate less than:_____

b) List the pathophysiological changes that occur as a consequence of insulin deficiency which explain the biochemical findings of hyperglycaemia, ketonaemia, acidosis and glycosuria. (4 marks)

Hyperglycaemia:_____

Ketonaemia:_____

Acidosis:_____

Glycosuria:_____

The results of her arterial blood gas are as follows:

pH	7.17
PCO_2	4.0 kPa
PO_2	12.1 kPa
HCO_3^-	<5 mmol/L
Base excess	−19.2 mEq/L
K^+	7.8 mmol/L
Na^+	129 mmol/L

c) Based on the arterial blood gas results above, what would be your immediate management? (1 mark)

_____

d) List the ECG changes that may be seen. (5 marks)

1. _____
2. _____
3. _____
4. _____
5. _____

e) List four other serious complications of DKA. (4 marks)

1. _____
2. _____
3. _____
4. _____

f) List the three endogenous ketone bodies. (3 marks)

1. _____
2. _____
3. _____

Question 4.

Diego, a 3-week-old boy born uneventfully at term, is brought by his mother to the Emergency Department with progressively worsening non-bilious vomiting, usually directly after a feed.

a) On assessment, Diego is severely dehydrated. List four clinical signs consistent with this class of dehydration. (4 marks)

1. _____
2. _____
3. _____
4. _____

A venous blood gas is taken, giving the following results:

pH	7.61
PCO_2	7.2 kPa
PO_2	11.0 kPa
Base excess	+30.1 mmol/L
Na^+	136 mmol/L
K^+	3.0 mmol/L
Cl^-	72 mmol/L

b) Interpret the venous blood gas. (1 mark)

_____

On the basis of the history and blood gas, you suspect a diagnosis of pyloric stenosis.

c) List four risk factors for developing pyloric stenosis. (4 marks)

1. _____
2. _____

3. _____

4. _____

d) List two additional features of the clinical examination consistent with a diagnosis of pyloric stenosis. (2 marks)

1. _____

2. _____

e) List two hormones secreted as a **direct** response to severe dehydration. (2 marks)

1. _____

2. _____

Despite the raised plasma pH, Diego's urine is found to be acidic.

f) Which hormone is responsible for this paradox? (1 mark)

_____

After 48 hours of intravenous rehydration, Diego's venous gas has normalised. The surgeons would like to perform a pyloromyotomy.

g) List six intra-operative and post-operative considerations **specific** to this age group and procedure. (6 marks)

1. _____

2. _____

3. _____

4. _____

5. _____

6. _____

Question 5.

Siobhan presents to the Emergency Department with a short history of painless vaginal bleeding. She is 38 weeks pregnant and is visiting family in England. She remembers being told about a low-lying placenta but has been unable to attend any follow-up antenatal clinics.

a) Describe the four grades of placenta praevia by their relationship to the internal cervical os. (4 marks)

Grade 1:_____

Grade 2:_____

Grade 3:_____

Grade 4:_____

b) Aside from a low-lying placenta, list five risk factors for placenta praevia. (5 marks)

1. _____

2. _____

3. _____

4. _____

5. _____

Following ultrasonography, Siobhan is told that her placenta is anterior and in a position that rules out normal vaginal delivery. Her observations are normal and her symptoms have now subsided. A decision is made to perform a caesarean section.

c) How may your anaesthetic differ for this procedure when compared to that of a low-risk elective caesarean section? (7 marks)

1. _____
2. _____
3. _____
4. _____
5. _____
6. _____
7. _____

Abnormal placental adherence describes the degree to which there is an invasion of chorionic villi into the myometrium because of a defect in the decidua basalis.

d) List the three forms of abnormal placental adherence (3 marks) in order of increasing incidence. (1 mark)

Least common:_____

Intermediate:_____

Most common:_____

Question 6.

Karen, a 65-year-old woman, is referred to pain clinic by her general practitioner. She has a 3-month history of pain on one side of her face in an area affected by a recent episode of shingles.

a) Name the virus that causes shingles. (1 mark)

_____

b) List the two most common sites for the shingles rash. (2 marks)

1. _____
2. _____

c) List three comorbidities which put patients at greater risk of developing **shingles**. (3 marks)

1. _____
2. _____
3. _____

d) List four risk factors for the development of **post-herpetic neuralgia** (PHN). (4 marks)

1. _____
2. _____
3. _____
4. _____

e) List six clinical features of PHN. (6 marks)

1. _____
2. _____
3. _____
4. _____
5. _____
6. _____

f) Regarding the pharmacological management, state a drug used to prevent PHN. (1 mark)

_____

g) List three first-line treatment options following the onset of PHN. (3 marks)

1. _____
2. _____
3. _____

Question 7.

Kevin, a 32-year-old man, is listed for excision of a parathyroid adenoma under general anaesthesia. The parathyroid adenoma was discovered following a series of investigations to identify the cause of Kevin's hypercalcaemia.

a) List six clinical features of hypercalcaemia. (6 marks)

1. _____
2. _____
3. _____
4. _____
5. _____
6. _____

b) Where are the parathyroid glands normally located? (2 marks)

_____
_____

c) Which investigation is used to locate the parathyroid adenoma pre-operatively? (1 mark)

_____

d) List four physiological effects of excess secretion of parathyroid hormone (PTH). (4 marks)

1. _____
2. _____
3. _____
4. _____

The patient's serum Ca^{2+} concentration on the day of surgery is 2.9 mmol/L. Your unit's policy is that surgery should proceed if the serum Ca^{2+} is below 3.0 mmol/L.

e) List two perioperative considerations in patients with moderate hypercalcaemia. (2 marks)

1. _____
2. _____

f) Following surgery, the patient becomes markedly hypocalcaemic. List four clinical features of acute hypocalcaemia. (4 marks)

1. _____
2. _____
3. _____
4. _____

g) The patient has a family history of hyperparathyroidism. Name an inherited endocrine condition which includes hyperparathyroidism. (1 mark)

Question 8.

You are asked to review Geraint, a 69-year-old man, in the Emergency Department. He has been vomiting violently throughout the night and has developed central chest pain. The general surgical registrar is concerned that he has Boerhaave syndrome (transmural oesophageal perforation).

a) List four clinical signs specific to a diagnosis of oesophageal perforation. (4 marks)

1. _____
2. _____
3. _____
4. _____

b) List four signs consistent with oesophageal perforation that may be seen on a CT scan. (4 marks)

1. _____
2. _____
3. _____
4. _____

A diagnosis of oesophageal perforation is made and an open oesophageal repair via a thoracotomy is planned.

c) State two considerations that may affect your drug choices during induction of anaesthesia. (2 marks)

1. _____
2. _____

d) List the two options for airway management in this case. (2 marks)

1. _____
2. _____

e) List two strategies that you would take to prevent lung injury during the case. (2 marks)

1. _____
2. _____

The procedure is difficult, and intra-operatively, the patient spends 8 hours in the lateral position.

f) List six complications of prolonged lateral positioning in this case. (6 marks)

1. _____
2. _____
3. _____
4. _____
5. _____
6. _____

Question 9.

Sarah, a 42-year-old woman, is listed for a laparoscopic cholecystectomy. Her body mass index (BMI) is calculated as 45 kg/m^2.

a) In which category of obesity would she be placed? (1 mark)

_____

At pre-operative assessment, the patient completes a STOP-BANG questionnaire which suggests she is at high risk of obstructive sleep apnoea (OSA).

b) Other than obesity, list four risk factors for the development of OSA in **all** patient groups. (4 marks)

1. _____
2. _____
3. _____
4. _____

c) List three health conditions that may result as a consequence of OSA. (3 marks)

1. _____
2. _____
3. _____

d) List four options that you would recommend to this patient for the management of her OSA. (4 marks)

1. _____
2. _____
3. _____
4. _____

The patient is established on OSA treatment and presents for a laparoscopic cholecystectomy.

e) List four physiological consequences of a raised intra-abdominal pressure as a result of pneumoperitoneum. (4 marks)

1. _____
2. _____
3. _____
4. _____

f) List four complications of the surgical positioning used when performing a laparoscopic cholecystectomy in this patient. (4 marks)

1. _____
2. _____
3. _____
4. _____

Question 10.

Matt, a 24-year-old man, is listed for a bimaxillary (combination of maxillary and mandibular) osteotomy.

a) List six perioperative airway concerns specific to bimaxillary osteotomy. (6 marks)

1. _____
2. _____
3. _____
4. _____
5. _____
6. _____

b) On examination, you notice that Matt has obstructed nasal passages. List three alternative methods of airway management for this case. (3 marks)

1. _____
2. _____
3. _____

c) List four techniques for minimising intra-operative blood loss during a bimaxillary osteotomy. (4 marks)

1. _____
2. _____
3. _____
4. _____

d) List three advantages for using total intravenous anaesthesia (propofol and remifentanil) for this case. (3 marks)

1. _____
2. _____
3. _____

e) List four precautions that you would take to reduce the risk of a retained throat pack. (4 marks)

1. _____
2. _____
3. _____
4. _____

Question 11.

Pete, a 22-year-old man with epilepsy and severe learning difficulties, is listed for a magnetic resonance (MR) scan of his brain under general anaesthesia.

a) Pete's parents ask you to provide premedication to avoid unnecessary distress during IV cannulation. List four pharmacological options. (4 marks)

1. _____
2. _____
3. _____
4. _____

b) Outline the physical principles of magnetic resonance imaging. (4 marks)

_____
_____
_____
_____

c) The MR scanner uses a superconducting magnet. What is superconductivity (2 marks), and how is it achieved (1 mark)?

Superconductivity:_____

_____

Achieved by:_____

The patient is sedated and the radiographers go through their safety checklist with his parents.

d) List four implanted ferromagnetic objects that may cause harm to the patient if subjected to the strong static magnet. (4 marks)

1. _____

2. _____

3. _____

4. _____

The patient is now anaesthetised and ready to enter the MR scanning room. A laryngeal mask airway (LMA) was chosen for airway management.

e) Which part of the LMA risks degradation of the MR image? (1 mark)

_____

f) Aside from the interaction between ferromagnetic objects and the strong static magnetic field, list four additional classes of hazards specific to the MR environment. (4 marks)

1. _____

2. _____

3. _____

4. _____

Question 12.

You are asked to assess Ash, a 32-year-old man who has been admitted to the Emergency Department after being trapped in a house fire. He has burns across his chest, abdomen and left arm. His estimated weight is 100 kg.

a) List five clinical features that would lead you to suspect a significant inhalational injury. (5 marks)

1. _____

2. _____

3. _____

4. _____

5. _____

b) What are the distinguishing features of the following degrees of burn injury? (3 marks)

First degree:_____

Second degree:_____

Third degree:_____

c) The ED registrar states that the patient has burns covering an estimated 30% body surface area (BSA). How has she come to this conclusion? (2 marks)

_____

_____

The ED nurse asks you to prescribe fluid for the patient. It has now been 1 hour since the patient was burnt.

d) What formula will you use to calculate this patient's intravenous resuscitation fluid? (2 marks) What will you prescribe? (2 marks)

Formula:_____

Prescription:_____

_____

_____

e) The ED registrar discusses the case with the regional burns centre. List three indications for transfer to a specialist burns centre. (3 marks)

1. _____

2. _____

3. _____

Although the patient's airway is currently patent, you remain concerned about an inhalational injury. You decide to intubate the patient prior to transfer to the regional burns centre.

f) List three management considerations **specific** to inhalational burn injury. (3 marks)

1. _____

2. _____

3. _____

Paper 5

Question 1.

On a routine visit to his general practitioner, James, a 59-year-old man, is suspected to have a pituitary adenoma. He is referred to an endocrinologist, who subsequently undertakes multiple tests. The insulin-like growth factor 1 (IGF-1) is raised, and the oral glucose tolerance test (OGTT) failed to suppress an endogenous hormone. Magnetic resonance imaging of the brain confirms a pituitary macroadenoma.

a) What is the visual field defect most commonly associated with a pituitary adenoma? (1 mark)

_____

b) What is the diagnosis in this case? (1 mark) List five further clinical features of this disease. (5 marks)

Diagnosis:_____

Clinical features:

1. _____
2. _____
3. _____
4. _____
5. _____

c) List six hormones secreted by the anterior pituitary and state the hormonal trigger for their release. (6 marks)

Table 5.1c **Hormones secreted by the anterior pituitary**

	Hormone	Trigger for release
1.		
2.		
3.		
4.		
5.		
6.		

James is listed for a trans-sphenoidal resection of his pituitary adenoma. During the procedure, the surgeon struggles to reach the adenoma and would like you to aid the descent of the pituitary gland into the operative field.

d) Name two techniques by which this can be achieved. (2 marks)

1. _____
2. _____

e) List two endocrine complications of pituitary surgery and two neurosurgical complications specific to trans-sphenoidal pituitary surgery. (4 marks)

Endocrine complications:

1. _____

2. _____

Neurosurgical complications:

1. _____

2. _____

f) Other than regular IGF-1 levels, what long-term follow-up will be needed after the procedure? (1 mark)

_____

Question 2.

Serena is a 63-year-old woman known to have age-related aortic stenosis. She is listed for an elective aortic valve replacement but has presented acutely with a fractured wrist. There is evidence of neurovascular compromise.

a) With the exception of age, state two causes of aortic stenosis. (2 marks)

1. _____

2. _____

b) State the valve area for each of the following classes of aortic stenosis severity. (4 marks)

Mild:_____

Moderate:_____

Severe:_____

Critical:_____

c) Serena has had a recent echocardiogram showing severe aortic stenosis. Give four anaesthetic principles you would employ during her general anaesthetic specific to her cardiac physiology and the reasoning behind them. An example has been completed for you. (8 marks)

Table 5.2c **Principles of the anaesthetic management of aortic stenosis**

Principle	Reasoning
Maintain intravascular volume	Ensure filling in face of raised left ventricular end-diastolic pressure

d) Serena's ECG shows left ventricular hypertrophy. What other abnormalities may be present on the ECG of a patient with severe aortic stenosis? (2 marks)

1. _____
2. _____

Two months later, Serena is admitted to hospital generally unwell and is diagnosed as having infective endocarditis.

e) State two major and two minor criteria (as per the modified Duke criteria) that may be used in the diagnosis of infective endocarditis. (4 marks)

Major criteria:
1. _____
2. _____

Minor criteria:
1. _____
2. _____

Question 3.

a) What percentage of major airway events reported to the National Audit Project (NAP) 4 originated during critical care intubation? (1 mark)

_____

b) List six patient-related factors that increase the risk of complications during the intubation of critical care patients. (6 marks)

1. _____
2. _____
3. _____
4. _____
5. _____
6. _____

The 'MACOCHA' score has been validated for airway assessment in critically ill patients.

c) List four of the components considered in the MACOCHA score. (4 marks) State the MACOCHA score that predicts a difficult intubation. (1 mark)

1. _____
2. _____
3. _____
4. _____

Score predicting difficult intubation:_____

d) List four indications for tracheostomy in critical care patients. (4 marks)

1. _____
2. _____
3. _____
4. _____

e) List four patient-related relative contraindications to percutaneous tracheostomy in critical care patients. (4 marks)

1. _____

2. _____

3. _____

4. _____

Question 4.

Ben, a 2-year-old boy with a history of severe cerebral palsy, presents for insertion of a percutaneous endoscopic gastrostomy (PEG) under general anaesthesia.

a) List two antenatal and two postnatal risk factors for the development of cerebral palsy. (4 marks)

Antenatal risk factors:

1. _____

2. _____

Postnatal risk factors:

3. _____

4. _____

b) List three clinical features that may occur in severe cerebral palsy related to the central nervous system (3 marks), and for each, state the anaesthetic implications. (3 marks)

Clinical feature 1:_____

Implication:_____

Clinical feature 2:_____

Implication:_____

Clinical feature 3:_____

Implication:_____

c) List two clinical features that may occur in severe cerebral palsy related to the gastro-intestinal system (2 marks), and for each, state the anaesthetic implications. (2 marks)

Clinical feature 1:_____

Implication:_____

Clinical feature 2:_____

Implication:_____

d) List two clinical features that may occur in severe cerebral palsy related to the respiratory system (2 marks), and for each, state the anaesthetic implications. (2 marks)

Clinical feature 1:_____

Implication:_____

Clinical feature 2:_____

Implication:_____

e) The patient takes regular baclofen to control muscle spasms. What are the mechanism and site of action of baclofen? (2 marks)

Mechanism of action:_____

Site of action:_____

Question 5.

You are asked to complete a telephone follow-up for Amali, a 32-year-old woman, who underwent an elective caesarean section under spinal anaesthesia 2 days ago. Following discharge, she has developed a severe headache.

a) List six clinical features of a post-dural puncture headache (PDPH). (6 marks)

1. _____
2. _____
3. _____
4. _____
4. _____
6. _____

b) List six other differential diagnoses of a post-partum headache. (6 marks)

1. _____
2. _____
3. _____
4. _____
5. _____
6. _____

c) What steps can you take when performing a spinal anaesthetic to reduce the risk of PDPH? (4 marks)

1. _____
2. _____
3. _____
4. _____

Due to childcare commitments, Amali is unable to present to the hospital for review as per your advice.

d) List four serious complications of untreated PDPH. (4 marks)

1. _____
2. _____
3. _____
4. _____

Question 6.

Heather, a 76-year-old woman with metastatic pancreatic cancer, is referred to the pain clinic by her general practitioner. Her current medication includes paracetamol, gabapentin, modified-release morphine and oral morphine. Your consultant is planning to perform a coeliac plexus block.

a) Which three sympathetic nerves unite to form the coeliac plexus? (3 marks)

1. _____
2. _____
3. _____

b) List two indications for a coeliac plexus block, other than for pancreatic malignancy. (2 marks)

1. _____
2. _____

c) Other than visceral pain, list two classes of cancer pain. (2 marks)

1. _____
2. _____

d) Using the posterior approach, describe how you would perform a coeliac plexus block. (6 marks)

_____
_____
_____
_____
_____
_____

e) List four procedural complications of coeliac plexus block (4 marks) and three complications resulting from sympathetic lysis. (3 marks)

Procedural complications:

1. _____
2. _____
3. _____
4. _____

Complications from sympathetic lysis:

1. _____
2. _____
3. _____

Question 7.

Doug, a 45-year-old man, presents to the Emergency Department having taken 80 of his antidepressant tablets. The emergency medicine physicians feel he is showing signs of serotonin syndrome.

a) What is serotonin syndrome? (1 mark)

_____

b) Name the triad of abnormalities seen in serotonin syndrome. (3 marks)

1. _____
2. _____
3. _____

c) List six of the Sternbach criteria for the diagnosis of serotonin syndrome. (6 marks)

1. _____
2. _____

3. _____

4. _____

5. _____

6. _____

d) Name four classes of drug which can trigger serotonin syndrome. (4 marks)

1. _____

2. _____

3. _____

4. _____

e) List four features of your management plan for the acute phase of serotonin syndrome. (4 marks)

1. _____

2. _____

3. _____

4. _____

f) How many serotonin receptor subtypes are found in humans (1 mark), and which of these is thought to be triggered in serotonin syndrome? (1 mark)

Number of receptor subtypes:_____

Receptor subtype triggered:_____

Question 8.

Nicola is a 58-year-old woman with a history of germ cell ovarian cancer. She is listed for a total abdominal hysterectomy and has undergone three cycles of neo-adjuvant chemotherapy.

a) Give one reason for the use of neo-adjuvant chemotherapy. (1 mark)

_____

b) List three classes of chemotherapy agent. (3 marks)

1. _____

2. _____

3. _____

c) For each of the systems listed below, give two specific systemic complications of chemotherapy relevant to anaesthesia. (12 marks)

Cardiac:

1. _____

2. _____

Respiratory:

1. _____

2. _____

Gastrointestinal:

1. _____

2. _____

Hepatic:

1. _____

2. _____

Haemopoietic:

1. _____

2. _____

Central nervous system:

1. _____

2. _____

d) As part of her neo-adjuvant chemotherapy, Nicola has been treated with bleomycin. List the techniques you would employ during her anaesthetic to reduce her risk of pulmonary toxicity. (3 marks)

1. _____

2. _____

3. _____

e) Which chemotherapy agent is most commonly implicated in the development of neurotoxicity? (1 mark)

Question 9.

Rhys, a 32-year-old pedestrian, has been struck by a passing car. He has an open left tibial fracture and abdominal pain. His observations in the resuscitation room are heart rate 126 beats/min, blood pressure 72/43 mmHg, respiratory rate 34 breaths/min, Glasgow Coma Score 15/15.

a) List six management priorities in the resuscitation of this patient prior to diagnostic imaging. (6 marks)

1. _____

2. _____

3. _____

4. _____

5. _____

6. _____

b) Name two investigations to help diagnose a splenic rupture. For each investigation, state the findings consistent with splenic rupture. (4 marks)

Investigation:_____

Findings:_____

Investigation:_____

Findings:_____

The investigations reveal a grade IV splenic injury, and the patient subsequently undergoes an open splenectomy.

c) List three immunological and two non-immunological functions of the spleen in an adult. (5 marks)

Immunological:

1. _____
2. _____
3. _____

Non-immunological:

1. _____
2. _____

d) Which three bacterial vaccinations should this patient receive, and what is the optimal timing for administration? (4 marks)

Vaccinations:

1. _____
2. _____
3. _____

Timing:_____

e) Which other long-term drug should be prescribed? (1 mark)

_____

Question 10.

Wilf, a 72-year-old man, attends pre-operative clinic. He is listed for a laparoscopic sigmoidectomy for cancer. He has Parkinson's disease.

a) What are the three clinical features that make up the classic triad of Parkinsonism? (3 marks)

1. _____
2. _____
3. _____

b) List a further clinical feature of idiopathic Parkinson's disease for each of the following classes. (4 marks)

Constitutional:_____

Motor:_____

Neuropsychiatric: _____

Autonomic:_____

c) What is the pathophysiology of idiopathic Parkinson's disease? (2 marks)

_____

Wilf has a complex drug regime for the management of his Parkinson's disease.

d) List three classes of drug that the patient might be taking, and give an example for each class. (3 marks)

1. _____
2. _____
3. _____

The surgeon is concerned because the patient will be nil by mouth for a period of time following his surgery.

e) Which two antiparkinsonian drugs can be administered parenterally? For each drug, give an advantage and a disadvantage. (6 marks)

Parenteral drug 1:_____

Advantage:_____

Disadvantage:_____

Parenteral drug 2:_____

Advantage:_____

Disadvantage:_____

f) List two antiemetics that are safe to use in Parkinson's disease. (2 marks)

1. _____

2. _____

Question 11.

a) What is the difference between capnometry and capnography? (2 marks)

_____

_____

Infra-red spectroscopy is the most common method of measuring carbon dioxide (CO_2) content in clinical practice.

b) Describe the physical principles behind infra-red spectroscopy. (3 marks)

_____

_____

_____

c) List four other methods of measuring carbon dioxide in its gaseous state. (5 marks)

1. _____

2. _____

3. _____

4. _____

5. _____

The diagram below is taken from a normal capnography trace.

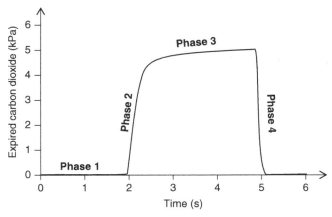

Figure 5.11d Normal capnography trace

d) Which gases (dead space and/or alveolar) are expired during phases 2 and 3? (2 marks) Indicate on the diagram where end-tidal CO_2 is determined. (1 mark)

Phase 2:

_____

Phase 3:

_____

e) List four roles of capnography during a cardiac arrest. (4 marks)

1. _____
2. _____
3. _____
4. _____

f) How can a Severinghaus electrode be used to measure the partial pressure of CO_2 in solution? (3 marks)

_____

_____

_____

Question 12.

A recent meta-analysis of studies of the utility of the Mallampati score in the prediction of a difficult airway found that it had a sensitivity of 60% and a specificity of 70%.

a) What is meant by the sensitivity of a clinical test (1 mark), and how is it expressed mathematically? (2 marks)

Sensitivity:_____

Described mathematically as:_____

_____

b) What is meant by the specificity of a clinical test (1 mark), and how is it expressed mathematically? (2 marks)

Specificity:_____

Described mathematically as:_____

_____

c) What is a meta-analysis? (2 marks)

_____

_____

d) What is a Forest plot? (1 mark) What do a square (2 marks) and a diamond (2 marks) represent?

Forest plot is:_____

Square represents:_____

_____

Diamond represents:_____

_____

e) List two types of bias to which a meta-analysis may be subject. (2 marks)

1. _____

2. _____

f) Regarding evidence-based recommendations, list the five 'levels of evidence', from the highest quality of evidence to the lowest quality of evidence. (5 marks)

1. (highest)_____

2. _____

3. _____

4. _____

5. (lowest) _____

Paper 6

Question 1.

Emma, a 40-year-old woman, is listed for excision of a vestibular schwannoma (acoustic neuroma).

a) List four commonly encountered clinical features of this condition. (4 marks)

1. _____
2. _____
3. _____
4. _____

The neurosurgeon is planning a translabyrinthine approach in the supine position as it is associated with a lower risk of damaging the seventh cranial nerve.

b) List four clinical features of seventh cranial nerve palsy due to neurosurgical trauma in this case. (4 marks)

1. _____
2. _____
3. _____
4. _____

c) List two other positions employed for excision of posterior fossa tumours. (2 marks)

1. _____
2. _____

The patient is anaesthetised, transferred onto the operative table and positioned supine with her head turned to the side. The surgery is expected to take more than 8 hours.

d) List four precautions you would take when positioning the patient. (4 marks)

1. _____
2. _____
3. _____
4. _____

e) List three strategies employed in neuroanaesthesia to avoid the patient coughing on extubation. (3 marks)

1. _____
2. _____
3. _____

f) The patient fails to wake following surgery. List three possible neurosurgical causes for decreased consciousness following posterior fossa surgery. (3 marks)

1. _____
2. _____
3. _____

Question 2.

Matthew, a 67-year-old man known to have chronic heart failure, is listed for an elective femoral endarterectomy.

a) Aside from advancing age, list three common causes of chronic heart failure within the Western world. (3 marks)

1. _____

2. _____

3. _____

Physiologically, the reduction in myocardial contractility seen in heart failure reduces stroke volume and increases both left ventricular end-diastolic volume and pressure.

b) State the two main re-modelling effects this has on the left ventricle. (2 marks)

1. _____

2. _____

c) The diagram below is of a normal left ventricular pressure–volume loop. Indicate the following:

1. Stroke volume, SV (1 mark)
2. Left ventricular end-diastolic pressure, LVEDP (1 mark)
3. End-systolic pressure–volume relationship (1 mark)

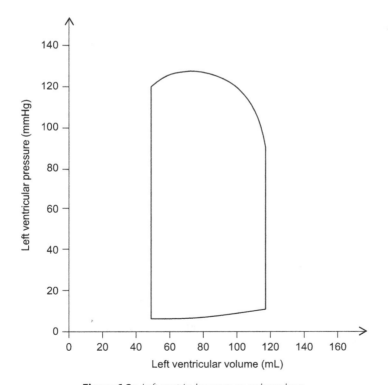

Figure 6.2c Left ventricular pressure–volume loop

On the same diagram, draw a loop to represent a chronically failing left ventricle with both diastolic and systolic impairment. Ensure that you indicate any changes in LVEDP or SV. You may assume that heart rate and systemic vascular resistance are unchanged. (3 marks)

d) The chronic reduction in cardiac output seen in heart failure invokes a neuroendocrine response activating which two systems? (2 marks)

1. _____
2. _____

e) List three classes of drug used to target the deleterious neuroendocrine response to chronic heart failure. (3 marks)

1. _____
2. _____
3. _____

f) Specific to **cardiac physiology**, give four techniques that you would employ during the patient's **intra-operative** management to preserve cardiac output and minimise myocardial workload. (4 marks)

1. _____
2. _____
3. _____
4. _____

Question 3.

You are asked to see Gareth, a 32-year-old man with known asthma. He has presented with increasing nocturnal dyspnoea over the last three nights and is now being treated in the resuscitation bay of the Emergency Department. A diagnosis of acute severe asthma is made.

a) List four drugs (with doses) used in the management of acute severe asthma. (4 marks)

1. _____
2. _____
3. _____
4. _____

b) List six clinical features of life-threatening asthma. (6 marks)

1. _____
2. _____
3. _____
4. _____
5. _____
6. _____

Gareth continues to deteriorate. You review him again and diagnose life-threatening asthma.

c) State four absolute and four relative indications for intubation and mechanical ventilation in life-threatening asthma. (4 marks)

Absolute indications:

1. _____
2. _____

3. _____
4. _____

Relative indictions:

1. _____
2. _____
3. _____
4. _____

d) The patient is intubated. What ventilator settings would you choose, and why? (4 marks)

Table 6.3d **Ventilator settings in life-threatening asthma**

	Ventilator setting	Reason
Respiratory rate		
Positive end-expiratory pressure (PEEP)		
Inspiratory: expiratory ratio		
Maximum inspiratory pressure (P_{max})		

e) Despite optimal ventilator settings, the patient does not improve. Name two other drugs that may be used in life-threatening asthma when the patient is on a mechanical ventilator. (2 marks)

1. _____
2. _____

Question 4.

Oscar is a 2-year-old boy brought to the Emergency Department by his parents following an episode of sudden coughing whilst eating 3 hours ago. On arrival, he has a respiratory rate of 30 breaths/min and evidence of a mild increased work of breathing. On auscultation, you note a localised wheeze on the right-hand side of the chest. Oxygen saturations are 95% in air.

a) What is the most likely diagnosis? (1 mark)

_____

b) Apart from increased respiratory rate, state four other features of an increased work of breathing in a child of Oscar's age. (4 marks)

1. _____
2. _____

3. _____
4. _____

c) Give four features that you may see on a chest radiograph with this diagnosis. (4 marks)

1. _____
2. _____
3. _____
4. _____

You opt to wait until Oscar is fasted before taking him to theatre.

d) State three advantages and three disadvantages of performing a gas induction with sevoflurane in oxygen for this case. (6 marks)

Advantages:

1. _____
2. _____
3. _____

Disadvantages:

1. _____
2. _____
3. _____

e) Name the drug and dose (in mg/kg) that you would use to anaesthetise the airway in Oscar's case. (2 marks)

Drug:_____
Dose:_____

f) Give three complications that may occur **post-operatively** specific to this case. (3 marks)

1. _____
2. _____
3. _____

Question 5.

You are called urgently to review Karen on the postnatal ward. She had an uneventful caesarean section earlier in the day but has collapsed on the ward with fresh blood per vaginam.

a) What are the four most common causes of primary postpartum haemorrhage? (4 marks)

1. _____
2. _____
3. _____
4. _____

b) The following table outlines the pharmacological management of obstetric haemorrhage. Complete the missing information. (7 marks)

Table 6.5b **Pharmacological management of obstetric haemorrhage**

Drug	Route of administration	Dose
Syntocinon	Intravenous	5 IU
	Intravenous	1 g
Carboprost (Hemabate)		
	per rectum	
Ergometrine		

c) List six non-pharmacological methods of managing obstetric haemorrhage. (6 marks)

1. _____
2. _____
3. _____
4. _____
5. _____
6. _____

d) In which common medical condition should the administration of carboprost be avoided? (1 marks)

_____

e) What are the two most common causes of secondary postpartum haemorrhage? (2 marks)

1. _____
2. _____

Question 6.

You are called to see Patrick, a 25-year-old man who has undergone a lower leg amputation following a crush injury 24 hours ago. He has been using patient-controlled analgesia (PCA) with intravenous morphine and was comfortable until 2 hours ago, when he started to experience severe pain.

a) Other than phantom limb pain (PLP), list four reasons why his pain control may have become inadequate. (4 marks)

1. _____
2. _____
3. _____
4. _____

b) How would you assess this patient? (3 marks)

_____

_____

_____

Alongside the morphine PCA, Patrick is prescribed regular paracetamol and ibuprofen.

c) List three further analgesic options to optimise his pain management. (3 marks)

1. _____

2. _____

3. _____

The acute pain is controlled, but you are asked to review Patrick 5 days later as he is developing symptoms of PLP.

d) What is the incidence of phantom limb pain following amputation? (1 mark)

_____

e) List three risk factors for the development of PLP in any amputee. (3 marks)

1. _____

2. _____

3. _____

f) State three peripheral mechanisms, two spinal cord mechanisms and one central mechanism responsible for the development of PLP. (6 marks)

Peripheral 1:_____

Peripheral 2:_____

Peripheral 3:_____

Spinal cord 1:_____

Spinal cord 2:_____

Central:_____

Question 7.

Alistair, a 6-year-old boy of Afro-Caribbean descent, is listed for an open reduction and internal fixation of a fractured radius. His sickle cell status is unknown.

a) List two pre-operative tests for sickle cell disease. (2 marks)

1. _____

2. _____

b) These tests establish that Alistair does have sickle cell disease (SCD). What is the Mendelian inheritance (1 mark), and what is the genetic abnormality? (2 marks)

Mendelian inheritance:_____

Genetic abnormality:_____

c) List five precipitants of sickling in SCD. (5 marks)

1. _____

2. _____

3. _____

4. _____

5. _____

d) What are the two pathophysiological consequences of red blood cell (RBC) sickling? (2 marks)

1. _____

2. _____

e) List eight clinical manifestations of SCD. (8 marks)

1. _____
2. _____
3. _____
4. _____
5. _____
6. _____
7. _____
8. _____

Question 8.

Victoria is due to undergo a caesarean section after failing to progress in the second stage of labour. An epidural was sited by your colleague earlier in the day and has been working well. Following assessment of the patient, you decide to top up the epidural in theatre with standard monitoring.

a) Apart from using a safe dose, list four steps that you can take to reduce the risk of local anaesthetic (LA) toxicity **during** performance of the block. (4 marks)

1. _____
2. _____
3. _____
4. _____

b) Explain, with reference to pharmacokinetics, why pregnant patients are at an increased risk of LA toxicity. (3 marks)

_____
_____
_____

c) In the table below, outline the maximum doses of the local anaesthetic agents shown. (4 marks)

Table 6.8c **Maximum doses of local anaesthetic agents**

Local anaesthetic	Maximum dose without adrenaline (mg/kg)	Maximum dose with adrenaline (mg/kg)
Lignocaine		
Bupivacaine		
Ropivacaine		
Prilocaine		N/A

d) List four patient-related risk factors for LA toxicity in non-obstetric patients. (4 marks)

1. _____
2. _____

3. _____

4. _____

Intravenous lipid emulsion (Intralipid®) should be administered as part of the management of LA-induced cardiac arrest.

e) Outline the details of the regimen that should be used for a **70 kg** female as described below. (4 marks)

Concentration of lipid emulsion (%): _____

Bolus dose (mL):_____

Initial infusion rate (mL/h):_____

Maximum cumulative dose (mL):_____

f) State an additional consideration regarding the duration of cardiopulmonary resuscitation in a patient with LA-induced cardiac arrest. (1 mark)

Question 9.

Stewart, a 42-year-old man, is to receive a cadaveric renal transplant. He currently undergoes haemodialysis three times weekly.

a) List four common causes of end-stage renal failure (ESRF) in the United Kingdom. (4 marks)

1. _____

2. _____

3. _____

4. _____

b) The patient arrives in the hospital and you perform your pre-operative assessment. List important aspects of your history (3 marks), clinical examination (2 marks) and pre-operative investigations (3 marks) specific to ESRF.

History:

1. _____

2. _____

3. _____

Clinical examination:

1. _____

2. _____

Pre-operative investigations:

1. _____

2. _____

3. _____

c) The patient has a left radial arterio-venous (AV) fistula. Name two perioperative implications of this. (2 marks)

1. _____

2. _____

d) List your intra-operative physiological goals to optimise the function of the transplanted kidney. (3 marks)

1. _____

2. _____

3. _____

e) In addition to paracetamol, list two options for post-operative analgesia in this case. (2 marks) Which analgesic would you avoid? (1 mark)

Analgesic options:

1. _____

2. _____

Avoid:

_____

Question 10.

Cath, a 64-year-old woman with a background history of hypertension, is listed for an elective laparoscopic cholecystectomy for gallstones.

a) Short-term control of blood pressure is under neural control. Where are the two high-pressure baroreceptors located? (1 mark)

_____

b) Describe the neural pathway involved in responding to an acute increase in blood pressure. (3 marks)

_____

_____

_____

c) Cath has primary (essential) hypertension. Define primary and secondary hypertension (1 mark), and list four causes of secondary hypertension. (4 marks)

Primary hypertension: _____

Secondary hypertension: _____

1. _____

2. _____

3. _____

4. _____

d) State end-organ complications of untreated hypertension on each of the following body systems. (6 marks)

Cardiac:

1. _____

2. _____

Renal:

1. _____

2. _____

Cerebrovascular:

1. _____

2. _____

On the day of surgery, Cath's blood pressure is found to be 215/115 mmHg. She last had her blood pressure measured by her GP when she was referred for surgery 5 months previously. On that occasion, it was measured as 170/105 mmHg.

e) What would be your initial management? (1 mark)

_____

f) If Cath had attended pre-operative clinic without any recent (within 12 months) blood pressure recordings, how high must the blood pressure be to lead you to postpone her operation? (1 mark)

_____

g) Bearing in mind Cath's community blood pressure of 170/105 mmHg, what would be your intra-operative blood pressure target, and why? (2 marks)

Target:_____

Reason: _____

h) What is the risk of stopping β-blockers in a hypertensive patient prior to their anaesthetic? (1 mark)

_____

Question 11.

Donald is a 62-year-old man who presents for a carotid endarterectomy (CEA) 8 days after experiencing a transient ischaemic attack (TIA). A carotid duplex scan demonstrated stenosis of his left internal carotid artery.

a) State the degree of stenosis at which a left CEA would be indicated. (1 mark)

_____

b) What is the recommended timing of surgery in relation to Donald's symptoms? (1 mark)

_____

The consultant anaesthetist with whom you are working suggests using a regional anaesthetic technique for the surgery.

c) List four advantages and four disadvantages of regional anaesthesia when compared to general anaesthesia, **specific** to CEA. (8 marks)

Advantages:

1. _____

2. _____

3. _____

4. _____

Disadvantages:

1. _____

2. _____

3. _____

4. _____

d) Your consultant plans to use a superficial cervical plexus block for this case. List two alternative local anaesthetic techniques which could be used for awake CEA surgery. (2 marks)

1. _____

2. _____

e) State how you would perform a superficial cervical plexus block using a landmark technique. (5 marks)

_____

_____

_____

_____

_____

In the post-anaesthetic care unit, Donald's blood pressure is 202/106 mmHg. On examination, he is confused, has a headache and has a right hemiparesis.

f) What is the diagnosis, and what is the underlying pathophysiology? (2 marks) What is your main management priority? (1 mark)

Diagnosis:_____

Pathophysiology:_____

Management:_____

Question 12.

Norman, a 78-year-old man, is listed for an Ivor Lewis oesophagectomy for cancer. He attends for a cardiopulmonary exercise test (CPET).

a) Regarding the metabolic equivalent of a task (MET), state the number of METs associated with each of the following. (4 marks)

Resting, fasted for >12 hours:_____

Walking at 2.5 mph on the flat:_____

Climbing two flights of stairs without stopping:_____

Jogging:_____

b) Other than CPET, list three **objective** methods of assessing exercise capacity. (3 marks)

1. _____

2. _____

3. _____

c) List four absolute contraindications to CPET. (4 marks)

1. _____

2. _____

3. _____

4. _____

d) List three cardiopulmonary responses to increased work on the cycle ergometer, demonstrated on the CPET nine-panel plot. (3 marks)

1. _____

2. _____

3. _____

e) List two CPET-derived variables, deficiencies of which are associated with poor post-operative outcomes. (2 marks)

   1. _____

   2. _____

f) Following the CPET, Norman's oxygen consumption is above baseline for a period of time. List four contributors to this 'oxygen debt'. (4 marks)

   1. _____

   2. _____

   3. _____

   4. _____

Paper 7

Question 1.

You are asked to review Catriona, a 28-year-old woman with myasthenia gravis who is listed for cardiothoracic surgery.

a) List four symptoms and two signs of myasthenia gravis. (6 marks)

Symptoms:

1. _____

2. _____

3. _____

4. _____

Signs:

1. _____

2. _____

b) What is the surgical procedure most likely to be? (1 mark)

_____

c) What are the two common proteins targeted by autoantibodies in myasthenia gravis? (2 marks)

1. _____

2. _____

d) Which subtype of immunoglobulin is produced? (1 mark)

_____

e) List three health conditions associated with myasthenia gravis. (3 marks)

1. _____

2. _____

3. _____

f) List three **classes** of drug that the patient might be prescribed pre-operatively to manage the symptoms of myasthenia gravis. (3 marks)

1. _____

2. _____

3. _____

Catriona is concerned about her risk of requiring post-operative ventilation.

g) Describe two methods you would consider to achieve intubation following induction of general anaesthesia that could reduce this risk. (2 marks)

1. _____

2. _____

Due to a miscommunication, the patient stops taking her medication pre-operatively and presents to the Emergency Department with features of a myasthenic crisis.

h) List two such features. (2 marks)

1. _____
2. _____

Question 2.

Mani is a 64-year-old man with a new diagnosis of lung adenocarcinoma. He is listed for a lobectomy of the right lung. He has a background history of chronic obstructive pulmonary disease.

a) Complete the following table regarding types of double-lumen tubes. (3 marks)

Table 7.2a **Types of double-lumen tubes**

Type of tube	Left- or right–sided, or both?	Carinal hook? (Yes/No)
White		
Robertshaw		
Carlens		

b) State two absolute indications for one-lung ventilation with a relevant example for each. (2 marks)

1. _____
2. _____

c) Mani has had a series of investigations prior to his surgery. What is the FEV_1 required to safely proceed with a lobectomy? (1 mark)

_____

Unfortunately, Mani's pulmonary function tests demonstrate that he does not have an adequate FEV_1 to be listed for surgery. He therefore undergoes a calculation of his predicted post-operative FEV_1 and predicted post-operative diffusion capacity.

d) What predicted percentage value for these tests would be considered acceptable to proceed with surgery? (1 mark)

_____

Mani's post-operative predicted ventilatory parameters are not adequate, and he is referred for cardiopulmonary exercise testing (CPET).

e) Which CPET parameter is primarily used for determining fitness for thoracic surgery (1 mark), and what value is required to be deemed suitable for surgery (1 mark), albeit as a high-risk candidate?

Parameter:

_____

Value:

_____

f) Hypoxaemia commonly occurs during one-lung ventilation. State three factors which impair hypoxic pulmonary vasoconstriction in the non-ventilated lung. (3 marks)

1. _____
2. _____
3. _____

During the surgery, Mani's oxygen saturation falls below 88%. You have checked the supply of gas and the position of the double-lumen tube, both of which are adequate. No secretions were present on suctioning of the ventilated lung.

g) List six steps that you would now take to manage the hypoxaemia. (6 marks)

1. _____
2. _____
3. _____
4. _____
5. _____
6. _____

h) List one potential advantage and one potential disadvantage of applying positive end-expiratory pressure (PEEP) to the ventilated lung. (2 marks)

Advantage:

_____

Disadvantage:

_____

Question 3.

Ajmal is a 47-year-old man who is referred to you by the medical team for consideration of critical care. He is known to have pulmonary hypertension (PH) and has presented with increasing exertional dyspnoea and pre-syncopal episodes precipitated by acute lower limb cellulitis.

a) What is the definition of PH? (1 mark)

_____

The World Health Organization (WHO) has classified PH into five categories.

b) List the five categories (one category has been completed for you). (4 marks)

1. Pulmonary arterial hypertension/idiopathic pulmonary hypertension
2. _____
3. _____
4. _____
5. _____

c) List four clinical signs of PH which you may identify when examining Ajmal. (4 marks)

1. _____
2. _____
3. _____
4. _____

d) List three ECG findings you may see with right ventricular hypertrophy. (3 marks)

1. _____
2. _____
3. _____

On reviewing his notes, you find he normally takes Tadalafil.

e) Explain the mechanism by which Tadalafil reduces pulmonary artery pressure. (3 marks)

_____
_____
_____

After discussion with your supervising consultant, Ajmal is admitted to the critical care unit.

f) Describe the principles of critical care management in the acutely unwell patient with pulmonary arterial hypertension. (5 marks)

_____
_____
_____
_____
_____

Question 4.

Sam is a 5-year-old boy weighing 20 kg who had a tonsillectomy earlier today. He is bleeding from the operative site and needs to return to theatre for haemostasis.

a) Define primary and secondary post-tonsillectomy bleeding. (2 marks)

Primary:_____
Secondary:_____

b) List two arteries that supply blood to the tonsils. (2 marks)

1. _____
2. _____

c) Aside from heart rate and blood pressure, list four further clinical signs that will indicate Sam's cardiovascular status. (4 marks)

1. _____
2. _____
3. _____
4. _____

Sam's previous anaesthetic chart reveals that he had a Cormack and Lehane grade 1 laryngoscopy.

d). Give two reasons why you would anticipate a potentially difficult intubation on return to theatre. (2 marks)

1. _____
2. _____

Sam has had a capillary blood gas which shows a haemoglobin of 89 g/L. You note that he is tachycardic and tachypnoeic. You opt to resuscitate him prior to anaesthesia.

e) State the type of fluid and the volume that you would give for initial resuscitation. (2 marks)

Fluid:_____

Volume:_____

f) There are two commonly described techniques for inducing anaesthesia in patients with post-tonsillectomy bleeding. Give both techniques, along with one advantage and one disadvantage for each. (6 marks)

Technique 1:_____

Advantage:_____

Disadvantage:_____

Technique 2:_____

Advantage:_____

Disadvantage:_____

g) Post-operatively, Sam's haemoglobin is noted to be 65 g/L. What volume of blood would you transfuse? (1 mark)

_____

h) What is the minimum length of time that Sam needs to remain in hospital following his return to theatre for bleeding tonsils? (1 mark)

_____

Question 5.

Kiran is a 27-year-old woman who is 32 weeks into her second pregnancy. She presents to the maternity unit with abdominal pain and an estimated blood loss of 500 mL per vaginum.

a) List five potential maternal complications of antepartum haemorrhage (APH). (5 marks)

1. _____

2. _____

3. _____

4. _____

5. _____

b) List five risk factors for placental abruption. (5 marks)

1. _____

2. _____

3. _____

4. _____

5. _____

Kiran continues to bleed, and her clotting profile shows significant abnormalities.

c) Define disseminated intravascular coagulation (DIC). (2 marks)

_____

_____

d) Apart from haemorrhage, list five other **obstetric** causes of DIC. (5 marks)

1. _____

2. _____

3. _____

4. _____

5. _____

e) Complete the following treatment goals for transfusion following massive obstetric haemorrhage. (3 marks)

Prothrombin (PT) ratio less than:_____

Platelet count greater than:_____

Fibrinogen concentration greater than:_____

Ionised calcium concentration greater than:_____

Temperature greater than:_____

Haemoglobin concentration greater than:_____

Question 6.

Siva is a 67-year-old man who presents to the Emergency Department with a fractured neck of femur following a mechanical fall. He has been seen by the orthopaedic team and listed for theatre later in the day. You are asked to assist in the management of his analgesia.

a) Name the four major nerves that supply the leg. (4 marks)

1. _____

2. _____

3. _____

4. _____

b) Aside from considering nerve blockade, list four recommendations made by the National Institute of Health and Care Excellence (NICE) regarding analgesia in a patient with a hip fracture. (4 marks)

1. _____

2. _____

3. _____

4. _____

You consent Siva for a fascia iliaca block.

c) List three other indications for a fascia iliaca block. (3 marks)

1. _____

2. _____

3. _____

An ultrasound machine is not available, so you decide to perform the block using a landmark technique.

d) Describe the 'stop before you block' process. (4 marks)

_____

_____

_____

_____

e) With reference to the relevant landmarks, describe where you would inject local anaesthesia during performance of a fascia iliaca block. (4 marks)

_____

_____

_____

f) Give the absolute contraindication specific to the performance of a fascia iliaca block. (1 mark)

_____

Question 7.

Ashraf is an 18-year-old man who presents to the Emergency Department 4 hours following a suicide attempt. He intentionally took 30 paracetamol tablets over the course of 2 hours.

a) Explain how an overdose of paracetamol causes hepatic damage. (4 marks)

_____

_____

_____

_____

b) List two clinical features of paracetamol overdose that may be evident within 24 hours. (2 marks)

1. _____

2. _____

c) When may you consider administering activated charcoal following a paracetamol overdose? (2 marks)

_____

_____

d) List four patient factors that increase the risk of hepatic injury following paracetamol overdose. (4 marks)

1. _____

2. _____

3. _____

4. _____

Ashraf is commenced on an infusion of N-acetylcysteine (NAC). You are asked to review him after he develops a tachycardia and a mild wheeze. On examination, an urticarial rash is noted. His oxygen saturations and blood pressure remain unchanged.

e) What is the likely diagnosis (1 mark), and how would you manage this situation? (3 marks)

Diagnosis:_____

Management:_____

_____

_____

Ashraf becomes unwell 48 hours later and is being considered for liver transplantation.

f) Name the prediction model most commonly used to identify liver transplant candidates in paracetamol hepatotoxicity (1 mark), and list three of the criteria. (3 marks)

Prediction model:_____

Criteria:

1. _____

2. _____

3. _____

Question 8.

Georgina, a 47-year-old woman, presented to her general practitioner with intermittent abdominal bloating and diarrhoea. She was referred for a CT scan, which demonstrated a carcinoid tumour in the small intestine with an isolated liver metastasis. She has been listed for elective resection of both lesions.

a) Other than the symptoms mentioned in the stem, give two further symptoms of carcinoid syndrome. (2 marks)

1. _____

2. _____

b) From what cell type do carcinoid tumours typically arise? (1 mark)

_____

c) List three substances secreted by carcinoid tumours. (3 marks)

1. _____

2. _____

3. _____

Two-thirds of patients with carcinoid syndrome will develop heart disease.

d) Which two heart valves are most commonly affected by carcinoid-related heart disease? (2 marks)

1. _____

2. _____

e) Georgina has been commenced on an octreotide infusion by her endocrinology team. Of which hormone is octreotide a pharmacological analogue? (1 mark)

_____

f) You opt to place a thoracic epidural to manage Georgina's post-operative pain. Give one advantage and one disadvantage of a thoracic epidural specific to the management of patients with carcinoid tumours. (2 marks)

Advantage:_____

Disadvantage:_____

g) Aside from AAGBI minimum monitoring standards, give three forms of monitoring that you would utilise in Georgina's surgery. (3 marks)

1. _____

2. _____

3. _____

h) During intra-operative handling of the tumour, Georgina develops signs of a carcinoid crisis. Apart from hypotension, list three clinical features that may be observed under anaesthesia in a carcinoid crisis (3 marks) and state the bolus dose of octreotide that you would administer for the management of this complication. (1 mark)

1. _____

2. _____

3. _____

Octreotide dose:_____

i) Despite the bolus of octreotide, Georgina remains hypotensive. Which vasopressor is safest to use, and which class of vasopressors should be used with extreme caution in patients with carcinoid tumours? (2 marks)

Safe:_____

Extreme caution:_____

Question 9.

Rhodri is a 42-year-old man listed for knee arthroscopy as a day-case procedure. He has a past medical history of type two diabetes mellitus.

a) When patients are referred for elective surgery, what is the HbA1c value above which surgery should be postponed to achieve better glycaemic control? (1 mark)

_____

b) List two further pre-operative tests that Rhodri will require. (2 marks)

1. _____

2. _____

Rhodri takes metformin, gliclazide and dapagliflozin. He is on the morning surgical list.

c) Complete the following table regarding the perioperative management of these drugs specific to day-case procedures. (6 marks)

Table 7.9c **Perioperative management of hypoglycaemic agents**

Drug	Mechanism of action	Dose on day of surgery (normal/halve/omit)
Metformin		
Gliclazide		
Dapagliflozin		

d) What is the recommended intra-operative blood glucose range for Rhodri, and how frequently should capillary glucose concentration be measured during the procedure? (2 marks)

Target:_____

Frequency:_____

e) State your pharmacological management (drug and dose) for the following intra-operative blood glucose abnormalities. (4 marks)

Blood glucose of 17 mmol/L:

_____

Blood glucose of 2.6 mmol/L:

_____

f) You are considering regional anaesthesia. Taking into account Rhodri's past medical history, state two advantages and two disadvantages of regional anaesthesia. (4 marks)

Advantages:

1. _____

2. _____

Disadvantages:

3. _____

4. _____

g) You opted to utilise dexamethasone during Rhodri's surgery. For what period of time should his blood glucose be monitored as a result of dexamethasone administration? (1 mark)

_____

Question 10.

Oliver, a 25-year-old man, is brought to the Emergency Department having thrown himself out of a second-floor window. He is known to suffer with schizophrenia and has attended his general practitioner twice in the last week with worsening delusional psychosis. You arrive 5 min after the patient is admitted into a resuscitation bay. His heart rate is 125 beats/min, blood pressure is 92/44 mmHg, and oxygen saturations are 92%. His Glasgow Coma Score (GCS) is 6/15.

a) What are the three components of the GCS? (3 marks)

1. _____

2. _____

3. _____

b) What is the most likely cause for his abnormal observations? (1 mark)

_____

You help to perform the primary survey. The airway is patent and breath sounds are vesicular. The abdomen and pelvis are bruised. There are no obvious long-bone fractures, and the GCS remains 6/15.

c) List three indications for intubation in this case. (3 marks)

1. _____

2. _____

3. _____

d) In addition to intubation, list your priorities for this case. (4 marks)

_____

_____

Oliver is found to have a vertical shear pelvic fracture, a base of skull fracture and cerebral contusions.

e) List four clinical signs which may be present as a consequence of the base of skull fracture. (4 marks)

1. _____
2. _____
3. _____
4. _____

f) List two clinical signs suggestive of urethral injury associated with a pelvic fracture. (2 marks)

1. _____
2. _____

g) Oliver remains in shock and ongoing pelvic bleeding is suspected. List three strategies to induce haemostasis. (3 marks)

1. _____
2. _____
3. _____

Question 11.

Kirsty, a 44-year-old woman, is listed for total thyroidectomy of a large multinodular goitre. She is clinically euthyroid and has no other past medical history.

a) List six aspects of the history and examination that are important to elicit **specific** to thyroidectomy. (6 marks)

1. _____
2. _____
3. _____
4. _____
5. _____
6. _____

b) List four pre-operative investigations indicated in this patient group. (4 marks)

1. _____
2. _____
3. _____
4. _____

Following a thorough pre-operative assessment, you do not anticipate any airway difficulties, and the patient is anaesthetised uneventfully. The size of the patient's thyroid gland makes the thyroidectomy a long and difficult procedure. Post-operatively, you are called urgently to the post-anaesthesia care unit, as Kirsty has become agitated and dyspnoeic. The recovery nurse thinks that Kirsty's neck has become more swollen; you suspect a neck haematoma.

c) List four other possible causes for an agitated, dyspnoeic patient specific to thyroid surgery. (4 marks)

1. _____
2. _____
3. _____
4. _____

d) The neck swelling continues to increase in size and the patient develops inspiratory stridor. List your management priorities in this case. (4 marks)

_____
_____
_____
_____

e) You manage to anaesthetise and intubate the patient, and the surgeon proceeds to re-explore the neck. During the procedure, the surgeon asks for a 'Valsalva manoeuvre'. State how you would perform a Valsalva manoeuvre in these circumstances and the purpose of doing so. (2 marks)

Valsalva manoeuvre:_____
_____

Purpose:_____

Question 12.

Vivek, a 39-year-old man, is listed for insertion of a vagal nerve stimulator.

a) List the three nuclei of the vagus nerve. (3 marks)

1. _____
2. _____
3. _____

b) List the immediate relations of the right vagus nerve in the neck at the level of the C6 vertebral body. (3 marks)

_____
_____
_____

c) List the immediate relations of the right vagus nerve in the thorax at the level of the T4 vertebral body. (3 marks)

_____
_____
_____

d) List six branches of the vagus nerve. (6 marks)

1. _____
2. _____
3. _____
4. _____

5. _____

6. _____

e) At what vertebral level does the vagus nerve pass through the diaphragm? (1 mark)

_____

f) List two indications for a vagal nerve stimulator. (2 marks)

1. _____

2. _____

g) A year later, Vivek presents for elective surgery unrelated to the vagal nerve stimulator. List two perioperative considerations specific to the nerve stimulator for this patient. (2 marks)

1. _____

2. _____

Paper 8

Question 1.

You are due to anaesthetise Brenda, a 15-year-old girl who is listed for a definitive correction of scoliosis.

a) Define scoliosis. (2 marks)

_____

_____

Adolescent scoliosis is most commonly idiopathic.

b) List four other causes of scoliosis. (4 marks)

1. _____
2. _____
3. _____
4. _____

c) The severity of Brenda's scoliosis has previously been defined using radiological imaging. What radiologically determined parameter is calculated to assess the severity of scoliosis, and at what value is surgical intervention indicated? (2 marks)

_____

_____

Your pre-operative assessment includes a comprehensive history, examination and airway assessment. Brenda tells you she has struggled to keep up with her peers recently when playing sport at school.

d) List two investigations of the respiratory system and two cardiac investigations that are indicated prior to surgery. (4 marks)

Respiratory investigations:

1. _____
2. _____

Cardiac investigations:

1. _____
2. _____

Brenda is worried about the risk of paralysis following the procedure. You explain that spinal cord monitoring will be used intra-operatively to help prevent irreversible damage.

e) Describe the neurophysiological monitoring used and how it indicates potential spinal cord injury. (4 marks)

_____

_____

_____

_____

f) List four pharmacological agents that may interfere with spinal cord monitoring. (4 marks)

1. _____
2. _____
3. _____
4. _____

Question 2.

Amare is a 69-year-old man listed for coronary artery bypass grafting. He has triple vessel disease that is not amenable to stenting.

a) Complete the labels (i–vii) on the following figure. (7 marks)

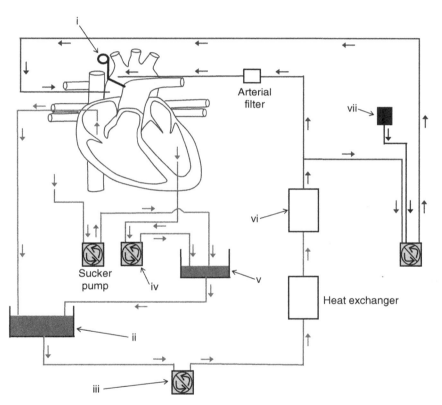

Figure 8.2a The cardiopulmonary bypass circuit. (Reproduced from D. Machin, C. Allsager. Principles of cardiopulmonary bypass. *Cont Edu Anaesth Crit Care Pain* 2006; **6**(5): 176–81

   i. _____
  ii. _____
 iii. _____
 iv. _____
  v. _____
 vi. _____
vii. _____

b) What is the standard dose of heparin given before initiation of cardiopulmonary bypass, and what activated clotting time (ACT) value should be attained prior to commencement of cardiopulmonary bypass? (2 marks)

Heparin dose:_____

Target ACT:_____

c) The surgeons are using cardioplegia for myocardial protection. State the mechanism by which the potassium-containing cardioplegia solution invokes diastolic arrest. (1 mark)

_____

d) State three physiological advantages of blood cardioplegia over crystalloid cardioplegia. (3 marks)

1. _____
2. _____
3. _____

e) Systemic hypothermia is a common feature of cardiopulmonary bypass. Give four physiological advantages and three physiological disadvantages of utilising systemic hypothermia during cardiopulmonary bypass. (7 marks)

Advantages:
1. _____
2. _____
3. _____
4. _____

Disadvantages:
1. _____
2. _____
3. _____

Question 3.

Justin, a 38-year-old man, is referred to the Intensive Care Unit with a possible diagnosis of Guillain–Barré syndrome (GBS).

a) What is GBS? (1 mark)

_____

b) List five clinical features of GBS. (5 marks)

1. _____
2. _____
3. _____
4. _____
5. _____

The neurologist reviews Justin and recommends immunoglobulin therapy.

c) List four side effects of immunoglobulin therapy. (4 marks)

1. _____
2. _____
3. _____
4. _____

d) What alternative treatment may be administered instead of immunoglobulin therapy? (1 mark)

_____

e) List six parameters or clinical indicators used to aid decision-making with regard to intubation in patients with GBS. (6 marks)

1. _____
2. _____
3. _____
4. _____
5. _____
6. _____

f) List three clinical features of GBS associated with a poorer overall outcome. (3 marks)

1. _____
2. _____
3. _____

Question 4.

You are called to the Emergency Department to assess Florence, a 2-year-old girl who presented with a 4-hour history of pyrexia and irritability. On examination, you notice a non-blanching rash. A presumptive diagnosis of meningococcal meningitis is made.

a) List four further clinical features of meningococcal meningitis. (4 marks)

1. _____
2. _____
3. _____
4. _____

b) What is the normal weight, heart rate, systolic blood pressure and capillary refill time for a child of this age? (4 marks)

Weight:_____

Heart rate:_____

Systolic blood pressure:_____

Capillary refill time:_____

c) Outline the initial management of this patient. (4 marks)

_____

_____

_____

_____

d) Which investigations will guide the care of this child? (2 marks) For each investigation, state the results that you would expect in this case. (4 marks)

Investigation 1:_____

Results:_____

_____

Investigation 2:_____

Results:_____

_____

e) Other than *Neisseria meningitidis*, name two common bacteria causing meningitis in this age group. (2 marks)

1. _____

2. _____

Question 5.

Megan, a 28-year-old primigravida, presents 2 days following an uneventful vaginal delivery. She is unwell with a temperature of 38.4°C and the obstetricians are concerned about puerperal sepsis.

a) List five risk factors for puerperal sepsis. (5 marks)

1. _____

2. _____

3. _____

4. _____

5. _____

b) List three reasons why regional anaesthesia is usually avoided in septic patients. (3 marks)

1. _____

2. _____

3. _____

c) List five common causes of non-obstetric sepsis in parturients. (5 marks)

1. _____

2. _____

3. _____

4. _____

5. _____

d) State the pathogen most commonly associated with maternal mortality. Name the two most common laboratory tests used in its identification. (3 marks)

Pathogen:_____

Laboratory test 1:_____

Laboratory test 2:_____

The Guideline for the Provision of Anaesthetic Services (GPAS) for an Obstetric Population (2018) describes standards of care for the acutely ill obstetric patient.

e) List four recommendations made regarding the care of the acutely ill obstetric patient. (4 marks)

1. _____

_____

2. _____

_____

3. _____

_____

4. _____

Question 6.

Deepak is a 74-year-old man listed for a left total shoulder replacement. He has a background of rheumatoid arthritis, and you have opted to supplement your general anaesthetic with a brachial plexus block.

a) From which nerve roots does the brachial plexus arise? (1 mark)

_____

b) Complete the following table regarding approaches to the brachial plexus and the level of the plexus at which the block is targeted. (6 marks)

Table 8.6b **Approaches to the brachial plexus**

Approach	Level of plexus
Interscalene	
	Cords

c) You opt to perform an awake interscalene block under ultrasound guidance prior to inducing anaesthesia. Please give four complications **specific** to interscalene block. (4 marks)

1. _____
2. _____
3. _____
4. _____

d) What length of block needle should be used for an interscalene block? (1 mark)

_____

e) Describe the anatomical location and vertebral level of the brachial plexus of relevance to an ultrasound-guided interscalene block. (2 marks)

_____
_____

f) Aside from reducing the risk of complications (including intraneural or intravascular injection), give three advantages of using an ultrasound-guided technique over an anatomical approach. (3 marks)

1. _____
2. _____
3. _____

g) Given his history of rheumatoid arthritis, state three reasons why performing an interscalene block may be more difficult in Deepak's case. (3 marks)

1. _____
2. _____
3. _____

Question 7.

Luis, a 25-year-old man, is brought into the Emergency Department after a high-speed road traffic collision. He has significant facial bleeding.

a) List six signs of airway compromise in facial trauma. (6 marks)

1. _____
2. _____
3. _____
4. _____
5. _____
6. _____

b) The patient is bleeding profusely from his mid face. Describe the three characteristic patterns of mid face fractures (Le Fort fractures). (3 marks)

Le Fort I_____

Le Fort II_____

Le Fort III_____

c) Give three methods to control the bleeding. (3 marks)

1. _____
2. _____
3. _____

The bleeding has stopped and no other injuries are identified. A CT scan demonstrates a Le Fort III fracture pattern. The following day, Luis is listed for surgical stabilisation of his facial fractures.

d) List two airway management options for the surgical correction of a Le Fort III fracture. (2 marks)

1. _____
2. _____

e) List six intra-operative anaesthetic considerations specific to this case. (6 marks)

1. _____
2. _____
3. _____
4. _____
5. _____
6. _____

Question 8.

Lynda, a 61-year-old woman, is listed for a total abdominal hysterectomy for uterine cancer. She has a history of chronic liver disease secondary to alcoholism but has been abstinent from alcohol for over 6 years.

a) Apart from alcohol abuse, list four causes of chronic liver disease. (2 marks)

1. _____
2. _____
3. _____
4. _____

b) Give two systemic effects of chronic liver disease on the body systems listed below. (8 marks)

Cardiovascular:
1. _____
2. _____

Respiratory:
1. _____
2. _____

Haematological:
1. _____
2. _____

Renal:
1. _____
2. _____

c) For the common anaesthetic drugs listed below, please detail the **specific** pharmacokinetic reason for reducing the dose in a patient with chronic liver failure. (4 marks)

Thiopental:_____
Rocuronium:_____
Morphine:_____
Alfentanil:_____

d) Give two options for Lynda's post-operative analgesia (appropriate for this type of surgery). State a **specific** disadvantage for each given her past medical history. (4 marks)

Analgesia option 1:_____
Disadvantage:_____
Analgesia option 2:_____
Disadvantage:_____

e) What is the estimated perioperative mortality (%) for patients with chronic liver disease in the following Child–Pugh classes? (2 marks)

Child–Pugh class A:_____
Child–Pugh class C:_____

Question 9.

You are reviewing Jen, an 82-year-old woman in pre-operative clinic who is listed for a total knee replacement. She has a history of chronic obstructive pulmonary disease and atrial fibrillation, for which she takes dabigatran.

a) State the mechanism of action for each of the following oral medications. (5 marks)

Warfarin:_____
Dabigatran:_____
Rivaroxaban:_____
Aspirin:_____
Prasugrel:_____

b) List four advantages and four disadvantages of direct oral anticoagulants (DOACs) when compared to warfarin. (8 marks)

Advantages:

1. _____
2. _____
3. _____
4. _____

Disadvantages:

1. _____
2. _____
3. _____
4. _____

c) Your supervising consultant suggests utilising spinal anaesthesia for the case. For each of the following oral medications, state the recommendations regarding cessation of the drug or acceptable drug activity level. (5 marks)

Warfarin:_____

Dabigatran:_____

Rivaroxaban:_____

Aspirin:_____

Prasugrel:_____

Before the date of surgery, Jen has a fall down the stairs. She is unconscious, and a CT scan identifies an intracranial haemorrhage.

d) List two methods for rapidly correcting the effects of dabigatran. (2 marks)

1. _____
2. _____

Question 10.

You review Stefan, a 64-year-old man, in the pre-operative anaesthetic clinic 1 month prior to planned colorectal surgery. Stefan is a lifelong smoker – you advise him to stop smoking and refer him to the smoking cessation service.

a) Give two reasons why smoking affects blood oxygen carriage. (2 marks)

1. _____
2. _____

b) List five perioperative complications of smoking related to the respiratory system. (5 marks)

1. _____
2. _____
3. _____
4. _____
5. _____

c) State four effects of nicotine on the cardiovascular system. (4 marks)

1. _____
2. _____
3. _____
4. _____

d) List three potential adverse effects of smoking cessation prior to surgery. (3 marks)

1. _____
2. _____
3. _____

e) List three benefits of Stefan abstaining from smoking in the 24 hours prior to surgery. (3 marks)

1. _____
2. _____
3. _____

f) Give three reasons why smokers are at an increased risk of thrombotic events in the perioperative period. (3 marks)

1. _____
2. _____
3. _____

Question 11.

a) Define ultrasound. (1 mark) Outline the principles by which ultrasound generates an image. (5 marks)

Definition:_____

Principles:_____

_____

_____

_____

_____

b) Explain how changing gain and frequency can alter the image produced. (2 marks)

_____

_____

c) List three forms of **acoustic artefact,** and for each, explain how it affects the image produced. (6 marks)

1. _____

_____

2. _____

_____

3. _____

_____

Echocardiography can be used to determine cardiac output by measuring the stroke volume and heart rate.

d) What two measurements are required to calculate stroke volume during echocardiography? (2 marks)

1. _____
2. _____

e) With the exception of echocardiography, list four uses of ultrasound in anaesthesia. (4 marks)

1. _____
2. _____
3. _____
4. _____

Question 12.

Bill, a 78-year-old man, has atrial fibrillation for which he takes warfarin. He is listed for a cataract operation as a day case under regional block.

a) List three benefits of day surgery to the patient. (3 marks)

1. _____
2. _____
3. _____

b) List three benefits of day surgery to the hospital. (3 marks)

1. _____
2. _____
3. _____

c) List three social factors which must be in place for a patient to be suitable for a day-case procedure. (3 marks)

1. _____
2. _____
3. _____

d) Bill's latest INR is 3.0. How would you manage Bill's perioperative anticoagulation? (1 mark)

_____

You plan to perform a sub-Tenon's block for this procedure.

e) Describe how you would perform a sub-Tenon's block. You may assume you have consented the patient, applied appropriate patient monitoring and have a trained assistant. (6 marks)

_____
_____
_____
_____
_____
_____

f) List four specific complications of regional anaesthesia of the eye. (4 marks)

1. _____
2. _____
3. _____
4. _____

Paper 9

Question 1.

Antonio, a 35-year-old man, presents for a laparoscopic cholecystectomy. He was diagnosed with myotonic dystrophy 10 years ago.

a) Define myotonic dystrophy (1 mark), state the underlying pathophysiology (1 mark) and Mendelian inheritance. (1 mark)

Myotonic dystrophy:_____

Pathophysiology:_____

Mendelian inheritance:_____

b) On pre-operative assessment, you notice that Antonio has the typical appearance of a patient with myotonic dystrophy – list two of these typical features. (2 marks)

1. _____
2. _____

c) List the clinical features of myotonic dystrophy related to the respiratory system (2 marks), cardiovascular system (2 marks), central nervous system (1 mark), gastrointestinal system (1 mark) and endocrine system. (1 mark)

Respiratory:

1. _____
2. _____

Cardiovascular:

1. _____
2. _____

Central nervous system:

1. _____

Gastrointestinal system:

1. _____

Endocrine system:

1. _____

The pre-operative echocardiogram demonstrated moderate left ventricular impairment and on further questioning, the patient's exercise tolerance is limited by breathlessness at a distance of 400 m.

d) List four considerations related to the induction of anaesthesia **specific** to myotonic dystrophy. (4 marks)

1. _____
2. _____
3. _____
4. _____

e) List four important aspects of intra-operative management **specific** to myotonic dystrophy. (4 marks)

1. _____
2. _____
3. _____
4. _____

Question 2.

Sukesh is a 73-year-old man who has an implanted pacemaker due to sick sinus syndrome. He is listed for an elective right hemi-colectomy for chronic diverticular disease.

a) The fundamental information about a pacemaker can be determined from its pacemaker code – what does each letter represent? (5 marks)

Letter 1:_____
Letter 2:_____
Letter 3:_____
Letter 4:_____
Letter 5:_____

b) What is meant by the sensitivity of a pacemaker? (1 mark)

_____

c) Aside from performing a pacemaker check, list three routine investigations you would request pre-operatively in a well patient with a cardiac implantable electronic device (CIED). (3 marks)

1. _____
2. _____
3. _____

d) In which three scenarios should re-programming of a CIED prior to anaesthesia/surgery be considered? (3 marks)

1. _____
2. _____
3. _____

e) Apart from monopolar or bipolar diathermy, state four devices or procedures that may produce electromagnetic interference of relevance to anaesthesia. (4 marks)

1. _____
2. _____
3. _____
4. _____

f) What is the commonest response of a permanent pacemaker (PPM) and an implantable cardioverter defibrillator (ICD) to the application of a magnet? (2 marks)

PPM:_____
ICD:_____

g) When applying external defibrillator pads, how far (in cm) from a CIED should the pads be placed? (1 mark)

_____

h) Aside from the risk of damage to the device itself, state one consequence of external defibrillation when the pads are positioned too closely to a CIED. (1 mark)   .

_____

Question 3.

Alice, a 39-year-old woman, presents to hospital with severe epigastric pain. Serum lipase is raised, and the general surgeons suspect acute pancreatitis.

a) What are the functions of the pancreas? (2 marks)

_____
_____

b) Aside from epigastric pain, list three presenting symptoms and signs of acute pancreatitis. (3 marks)

1. _____
2. _____
3. _____

c) List five common causes of acute pancreatitis. (5 marks)

1. _____
2. _____
3. _____
4. _____
5. _____

d) List four strong indicators for a critical care admission in a patient with severe acute pancreatitis (SAP). (4 marks)

1. _____
2. _____
3. _____
4. _____

e) In which two situations may surgical intervention be helpful in managing SAP? (2 marks)

1. _____
2. _____

f) When should enteral nutrition be commenced? (1 mark)

_____

g) List three benefits of enteral nutrition over parenteral nutrition in SAP. (3 marks)

1. _____
2. _____
3. _____

Question 4.

Miles is a 1-day-old neonate born at 38 weeks' gestation with a birth weight of 2.0 kg. He was antenatally diagnosed with an isolated tracheoesophageal fistula (TOF) and is listed for urgent repair.

a) What is the incidence of tracheoesophageal fistula? (1 mark)

_____

Tracheoesophageal fistulas are often associated with other congenital anomalies.

b) List three congenital anomalies associated with TOF. (3 marks)

1. _____
2. _____
3. _____

c) State three important aspects of the induction and intubation **specific** to Miles' condition. (3 marks)

1. _____
2. _____
3. _____

d) As a neonate, Miles will have a number of physiological differences from adults. For each of the body systems listed below, list three **physiological** differences of neonates when compared to adults. (9 marks)

Respiratory:

1. _____
2. _____
3. _____

Cardiovascular:

1. _____
2. _____
3. _____

Haematological:

1. _____
2. _____
3. _____

e) List three reasons why neonates are more vulnerable to hypothermia. (3 marks)

1. _____
2. _____
3. _____

f) As a 1-day-old neonate, what is Miles' 24-hour fluid maintenance requirement (in mL/kg)? (1 mark)

_____

Question 5.

a) What are the primary functions of the placenta? (3 marks)

1. _____
2. _____
3. _____

b) List the four main mechanisms of drug transfer across the placenta. (4 marks)

1. _____
2. _____

3. _____

4. _____

c) List six factors affecting drug transfer across the placenta. (6 marks)

1. _____

2. _____

3. _____

4. _____

5. _____

6. _____

d) With reference to the relevant pharmacokinetics, explain why bupivacaine administered via an epidural to the mother may accumulate in the foetus. (4 marks)

_____

_____

_____

_____

e) Explain the potential foetal adverse effect of administering neostigmine combined with glycopyrrolate during pregnancy. (2 marks) How might you mitigate this effect when using neostigmine? (1 mark)

_____

_____

_____

Question 6.

You have been asked to review Simona on the delivery suite. Following a low-risk pregnancy she went into spontaneous labour earlier in the day. She has been struggling with pain and has been transferred to the delivery suite for consideration of additional analgesia.

a) Describe the causes and pathways of visceral (3 marks) and somatic pain (3 marks) in labour.

Visceral:_____

_____

_____

Somatic:_____

_____

_____

After discussing the options available with Simona, she opts for an epidural.

b) State the anatomical boundaries of the epidural space. (4 marks)

Anterior:_____

Posterior:_____

Superior:_____

Inferior:_____

After siting the epidural successfully, you start an epidural infusion of bupivacaine and fentanyl.

c) State three mechanisms by which epidural opioids exert their effects. (3 marks)

1. _____
2. _____
3. _____

d) List three benefits of using epidural fentanyl over epidural diamorphine. (3 marks)

1. _____
2. _____
3. _____

The epidural is continued following delivery to aid the suturing of a first-degree tear. The midwife asks you to review Simona, as she is concerned about increasing leg weakness.

e) The table below outlines the Bromage scale of motor blockade. Complete the missing criteria. (2 marks)

Table 9.6e **Bromage scale of motor blockade**

Grade	Criteria	Degree of block
1	Free movement of legs and feet	Nil
2		Partial
3		Almost complete
4	Unable to move legs or feet	Complete

f) On assessment, Simona has a Bromage grade 4 leg weakness. Outline the steps you would take, including when you would request an urgent magnetic resonance imaging (MRI) scan. (2 marks)

Steps:_____

When to request MRI scan:_____

Question 7.

Davinder is a 57-year-old man who is listed for a transurethral resection of prostate (TURP) for benign prostatic hypertrophy. After discussion with the patient, you decide on spinal anaesthesia.

a) Apart from avoiding the adverse effects of general anaesthesia, list four advantages of using a neuraxial technique **specific** to this case. (4 marks)

1. _____
2. _____
3. _____
4. _____

b) From which nerve roots does the sympathetic and parasympathetic innervation to the prostate gland arise? (2 marks)

Sympathetic:_____

Parasympathetic:_____

c) What is the optimum spinal block height for this case, and why? (1 mark)

Block height:_____

Reason:_____

Glycine 1.5% is the irrigation fluid that is used for the procedure.

d) List four features of the **ideal** irrigation fluid. (4 marks)
   1. _____
   2. _____
   3. _____
   4. _____

e) List four factors that **increase** the rate of absorption of irrigation fluid during surgery. (4 marks)
   1. _____
   2. _____
   3. _____
   4. _____

Towards the end of the procedure, Davinder becomes restless and complains of a headache, breathlessness and a burning sensation in his hands and face. He requires oxygen via nasal cannulae to maintain oxygen saturations, and his systolic blood pressure has fallen by 20%. He becomes increasingly confused, and you believe he has transurethral resection (TUR) syndrome.

f) What immediate action should be taken? (1 mark)

_____

g) Explain the pathophysiological mechanisms behind two further clinical features of TUR syndrome. (4 marks)

Clinical feature 1:_____
Pathophysiology:_____
Clinical feature 2:_____
Pathophysiology:_____

Question 8.

William, a 25-year-old man, is admitted to hospital following a road traffic collision in which he sustained a left femoral fracture. A day later, he is listed for an intra-medullary nailing of the fracture but seems to be exhibiting symptoms consistent with fat embolism.

a) Which three body systems are implicated in the classic clinical triad of fat embolism? (3 marks)
   1. _____
   2. _____
   3. _____

b) List three of Gurd's minor criteria for a diagnosis of fat embolus. (3 marks)
   1. _____
   2. _____
   3. _____

c) What are the two proposed theories for the pathophysiology of fat embolism? (2 marks) For each, briefly describe the proposed mechanism. (4 marks)

Theory 1:_____
Mechanism:_____

Theory 2:_____

Mechanism:_____

d) Aside from long-bone fractures, state two trauma-related injuries associated with the development of fat embolism. (2 marks)

1. _____
2. _____

e) State two non-trauma-related conditions associated with the development of fat embolism. (2 marks)

1. _____
2. _____

f) Give two management techniques that may reduce the incidence of fat embolism in at-risk trauma patients. (2 marks)

1. _____
2. _____

g) State a common abnormality found on the full blood count of patients known to have a fat embolus. (1 mark)

_____

h) What is the estimated mortality of fat embolism syndrome? (1 mark)

_____

Question 9.

a) List three clinical uses of nitrous oxide (N_2O). (3 marks)

1. _____
2. _____
3. _____

b) State the molecular weight, boiling point and minimum alveolar concentration of N_2O (include units). (3 marks)

Molecular weight:_____

Boiling point:_____

Minimum alveolar concentration:_____

c) How is nitrous oxide produced and stored? Include the equation for nitrous oxide production in your answer. (4 marks)

_____

_____

_____

_____

d) What are the pharmacodynamic effects of N_2O on the respiratory and cardiovascular systems? (4 marks)

Respiratory system:_____

Cardiovascular system:_____
_____

e) List six adverse effects of N_2O. (6 marks)

1. _____
2. _____
3. _____
4. _____
5. _____
6. _____

Question 10.

Franklin is a 26-year-old Foundation Year 2 doctor about whom concerns have been raised regarding possible substance misuse.

a) Define substance abuse. (1 mark)

_____

b) Define dependence and tolerance. (2 marks)

Dependence:_____

Tolerance:_____

c) List the most common drugs abused by **doctors** in training. (3 marks)

1. _____
2. _____
3. _____

d) List four **general** risk factors for developing substance abuse disorders (4 marks), and three risk factors **specific** to doctors. (3 marks)

General risk factors:

1. _____
2. _____
3. _____
4. _____

Risk factors specific to doctors:

1. _____
2. _____
3. _____

e) List three potential consequences of substance abuse by a doctor in training. (3 marks)

1. _____
2. _____
3. _____

f) Define relapse (1 mark), and list three predictors for a relapse. (3 marks)

Definition:_____

Predictors:

1. _____

2. _____

3. _____

Question 11.

Edward is an 82-year-old man who is listed for an emergency laparotomy for a small bowel obstruction. He has a past medical history of ischaemic heart disease and his echocardiogram demonstrates moderate diastolic impairment. You have opted to utilise cardiac output monitoring as part of your anaesthetic.

a) What is considered the 'gold standard' cardiac output monitor? (1 mark)

_____

b) State two intra-operative advantages of utilising a cardiac output monitor. (2 marks)

1. _____

2. _____

c) Define the following terms related to cardiac output monitoring. (3 marks)

Preload:_____

Afterload:_____

Mean arterial pressure:_____

You have opted to use an oesophageal Doppler during Edward's anaesthesia and surgery.

d) Define the Doppler effect. (1 mark)

_____

e) Describe the process through which the oesophageal Doppler probe determines cardiac output. (5 marks)

_____

_____

_____

_____

_____

f) Complete the following table regarding the common variables produced by the oesophageal Doppler probe. (4 marks)

Table 9.11f **Oesophageal Doppler variables**

Variable	Description	Normal value (healthy adult)
Flow time corrected (FTc)		
Peak velocity (PV)		

g) List four disadvantages of using an oesophageal Doppler probe. (4 marks)

1. _____

2. _____
3. _____
4. _____

Question 12.

a) List three advantages and three disadvantages of point-of-care (POC) coagulation testing. (6 marks)

Advantages:
1. _____
2. _____
3. _____

Disadvantages:
1. _____
2. _____
3. _____

b) The diagram below shows a normal POC coagulation trace. Explain what each label represents physiologically. (4 marks)

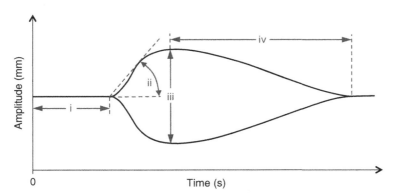

Figure 9.12b POC coagulation trace

i. _____
ii. _____
iii. _____
iv. _____

c) In the following table, indicate the most appropriate blood product or drug that should be given to help correct the abnormality. (4 marks)

Table 9.12c **POC coagulation trace abnormalities**

Abnormality	Response
Increased (i)	
Decreased (ii)	
Decreased (iii)	
Decreased (iv)	

d) Thromboelastography (TEG®) is a commonly used POC coagulation device. Explain how this device works. (5 marks)

_____

_____

_____

_____

_____

e) What volume of blood is required for POC coagulation testing? (1 mark)

_____

Paper 10

Question 1.

Eliza, an 8-year-old girl, is unwell and is brought into the Emergency Department (ED) by a paramedic crew. On arrival at the ED, she has a tonic-clonic seizure.

a) List four causes of seizures in this age group. (4 marks)

1. _____
2. _____
3. _____
4. _____

b) List three seizure types other than tonic-clonic. (3 marks)

1. _____
2. _____
3. _____

c) Outline your initial patient management. (3 marks)

1. _____
2. _____
3. _____

d) State your **pharmacological** management (with per kilogram doses) of this situation according to the following time frames. (6 marks)

At 5 min:

1. _____
or 2._____

At 15 min:

_____

At 25 min:

1. _____
or 2._____

At 45 min:

_____

e) Which endotracheal tube (ETT) size would you use for this child? (1 mark)

_____

Eliza is now successfully intubated, and you need to transfer her for a CT scan. Three full oxygen cylinders of different sizes are available.

f) What is the volume of oxygen stored within each? (3 marks)

Size CD _____
Size E _____
Size F _____

Question 2.

Bob is a 79-year-old man with known coronary artery disease. The surgical team would like to perform off-pump coronary artery bypass grafting.

a) List four features of a patient's past medical history that might make an off-pump procedure preferable. (4 marks)

1. _____
2. _____
3. _____
4. _____

b) What is the target activated clotting time (ACT) for off-pump coronary artery bypass graft surgery? (1 mark)

_____

c) In order to work on the posterior and lateral surfaces of the heart, it must be lifted vertically out of the pericardial sac. Give two physiological reasons why this may cause haemodynamic compromise. (2 marks)

1. _____
2. _____

d) A decrease in mean arterial blood pressure is common during off-pump coronary artery bypass. List three intra-operative strategies used to restore blood pressure to normal limits. (3 marks)

1. _____
2. _____
3. _____

Tachycardia is deleterious during off-pump bypass surgery owing to the consequent increase in myocardial oxygen demand; esmolol or verapamil is often used to decrease myocardial oxygen demand.

e) Complete the following table regarding these two drugs. (6 marks)

Table 10.2e. **Drugs used in the management of intra-operative tachycardia**

Drug	Specific receptor activity	Metabolism	Affected phase of pacemaker action potential
Esmolol			
Verapamil			

f) State four reasons why off-pump coronary bypass surgery is considered more 'cost-effective' than cardiopulmonary bypass. (4 marks)

1. _____
2. _____
3. _____
4. _____

Question 3.

You are asked to review Johnny, a 56-year-old man, on the respiratory ward. He presented to hospital 2 days ago with acute severe pneumonia. An arterial blood gas reveals type 1 respiratory failure, and you believe he has acute respiratory distress syndrome (ARDS).

a) List four components of the Berlin definition of ARDS. (4 marks)

1. _____
2. _____
3. _____
4. _____

b) List four ventilatory strategies used to prevent further lung injury whilst maintaining oxygenation. (4 marks)

1. _____
2. _____
3. _____
4. _____

Despite optimal management, Johnny's oxygenation continues to decline, and a decision is made to reposition him into the prone position.

c) List three effects of the prone position on the respiratory system that aid oxygenation. (3 marks)

1. _____
2. _____
3. _____

Two days later, Johnny is discussed at the multi-disciplinary meeting, and it is suggested that he be considered for extracorporeal membrane oxygenation (ECMO). You are asked to calculate his Murray score.

d) List the four components used to calculate the Murray score. (4 marks)

1. _____
2. _____
3. _____
4. _____

e) List four contraindications to ECMO. (4 marks)

1. _____
2. _____
3. _____
4. _____

f) What type of ECMO circuit is most commonly used to facilitate gas exchange when cardiac function is preserved? (1 mark)

Question 4.

Olivia is a 3-year-old girl weighing 15 kg who is listed for elective day-case strabismus surgery. She has no other past medical history of note, takes no regular medication and has no drug allergies.

a) Name two syndromes associated with strabismus. (2 marks)

_____

_____

b) On clinical examination, you hear a cardiac murmur. List three clinical features of an innocent murmur. (3 marks)

1. _____
2. _____
3. _____

c) You plan to administer the following pre- and intra-operative medication. Complete the table. (5 marks)

Table 10.4c. **Paediatric drug doses**

Drug	Dose (units/kg)	Route
Paracetamol		Oral
Ibuprofen		Oral
Glycopyrrolate		Intravenous
Ondansetron		Intravenous
Dexamethasone		Intravenous

d) During her strabismus surgery, Olivia suddenly becomes bradycardic. Name the reflex causing this bradycardia, and state the specific afferent and efferent nerves involved. (3 marks)

Reflex:_____

Afferent limb:_____

Efferent limb:_____

e) Olivia has met the criteria for day-case surgery. List four patient-related factors and three social factors that would exclude a paediatric patient from day-case surgery. (7 marks)

Patient-related factors:

1. _____
2. _____
3. _____
4. _____

Social factors:

1. _____
2. _____
3. _____

Question 5.

Hazra is a 34-year-old primigravida who is 38 weeks pregnant. She presents to the maternity unit with a 1-week history of increasing shortness of breath, ankle swelling and fatigue.

a) Which three criteria must be met to make a diagnosis of peripartum cardiomyopathy (PPCM)? (3 marks)

1. _____
2. _____
3. _____

b) List three changes you may see on an ECG in a normal pregnancy. (3 marks)

1. _____
2. _____
3. _____

c) List five risk factors for PPCM. (5 marks)

1. _____
2. _____
3. _____
4. _____
5. _____

Hazra undergoes a caesarean section under combined spinal–epidural anaesthesia.

d) List five **principles** of intra-operative management in this case. (5 marks)

1. _____
2. _____
3. _____
4. _____
5. _____

e) For each of the following uterotonics, state two deleterious effects that may occur in patients with PPCM. (4 marks)

Oxytocin:

1. _____
2. _____

Ergometrine:

1. _____
2. _____

Question 6.

Ada, a 62-year-old woman, is listed for excision of a large ovarian mass through a lower-midline laparotomy. She has a history of chronic back pain, and her regular medication includes pregabalin 150 mg bd and modified-release oxycodone 40 mg bd. She has recently had a spinal cord stimulator (SCS) inserted.

a) List two indications for SCS insertion. (2 marks)

1. _____
2. _____

b) List two contraindications to spinal cord stimulator insertion. (2 marks)

   1. _____

   2. _____

c) What are the two component parts of a spinal cord stimulator? (2 marks)

   1. _____

   2. _____

d) State two perioperative implications of the spinal cord stimulator. (2 marks)

   1. _____

   2. _____

e) List four methods that utilise local anaesthesia which may be used to manage this patient's post-operative pain. (4 marks)

   1. _____

   2. _____

   3. _____

   4. _____

The surgery was complicated by bowel injury, and a primary anastomosis was performed. Despite administering intra-operative paracetamol and parecoxib and using a regional anaesthetic technique, Ada has severe pain in the post-anaesthesia care unit.

f) List, **with doses**, three non-opioid analgesics which could be used in this case. (3 marks)

   1. _____

   2. _____

   3. _____

g) Ada is expected to be nil by mouth for the next 2 days. List three early symptoms or signs of opioid withdrawal. (3 marks)

   1. _____

   2. _____

   3. _____

h) What are the ratios of conversion from oral oxycodone into oral morphine and oral morphine into intravenous morphine? (2 marks)

Oral oxycodone : oral morphine_____

Oral morphine : intravenous morphine_____

Question 7.

Derrick, a 68-year-old man, is listed for a laparoscopic anterior resection for a recently diagnosed bowel cancer. He has a past medical history of hypertension.

a) List two cytokines thought to initiate the surgical stress response. (2 marks)

   1. _____

   2. _____

b) For each of the following hormones, state two physiological effects of their release related to the surgical stress response. (4 marks)

Cortisol:

1. _____

2. _____

Growth hormone:

3. _____

4. _____

A pre-operative full blood count has revealed a microcytic anaemia with a haemoglobin of 107 g/L. Derrick's surgery is listed for 6 weeks' time.

c) What are the two treatment options? Give one advantage and one disadvantage for each option. (6 marks)

Option 1:_____

Advantage:_____

Disadvantage:_____

Option 2:_____

Advantage:_____

Disadvantage:_____

Derrick is admitted on the day of surgery as per the enhanced recovery pathway. Once he is anaesthetised, you insert an oesophageal Doppler probe.

d) How would you use this cardiac output monitor for goal-directed fluid therapy? (3 marks)

_____

_____

_____

e) Aside from goal-directed fluid therapy, state two further elements of your intra-operative care for Derrick in the context of an enhanced recovery pathway. (2 marks)

1. _____

2. _____

f) State three features of post-operative care for a patient, such as Derrick, on an enhanced recovery pathway. (3 marks)

1. _____

2. _____

3. _____

Question 8.

John is a 31-year-old cyclist who has suffered major injuries following a road traffic collision. On arrival at the Emergency Department, he is noted to be tachycardic and hypotensive with a tense abdomen. A trauma CT reveals a ruptured spleen and multiple liver lacerations. He is listed for an emergency laparotomy, and you have activated the major haemorrhage protocol.

a) Give a definition for 'major haemorrhage' and a definition for 'massive transfusion'. (2 marks)

Major haemorrhage:_____

Massive transfusion:_____

b) List the three components of the lethal triad of trauma (3 marks), and for each component, give one deleterious consequence **specific** to the coagulation process. (3 marks)

Table 10.8b. **Lethal triad of trauma**

Component	Consequence

Intra-operatively, John continues to bleed, and you administer blood products.

c) For each listed blood product, state the target value which would indicate adequate transfusion. (4 marks)

Packed red blood cells:_____

Fresh frozen plasma:_____

Cryoprecipitate:_____

Platelets:_____

d) Using the sub-headings provided, list the complications of **massive transfusion**. (6 marks)

Transfusion reactions:

1. _____

2. _____

Immunological reactions:

1. _____

2. _____

Metabolic complications:

1. _____

2. _____

e) What effect does tranexamic acid have on the coagulation cascade, and what dose would you use in an adult major trauma patient? (2 marks)

Effect:_____

Dose:_____

Question 9.

You attend the departmental morbidity and mortality meeting where recent critical incidents are reviewed. Two corneal abrasions are reported, and preventative steps are discussed.

a) List three causes of corneal abrasion under general anaesthesia (3 marks) and three physical measures you can take to help prevent corneal abrasions from occurring. (3 marks)

Causes of corneal abrasion:

1. _____

2. _____

3. _____

Physical prevention measures:

1. _____

2. _____

3. _____

Liz discussed a case of common peroneal nerve palsy after prolonged surgery in the lithotomy position which had led to legal action.

b) List three clinical features of common peroneal nerve palsy. (3 marks)

1. _____

2. _____

3. _____

c) Aside from common peroneal nerve injury, list the two most common nerve injuries associated with general anaesthesia. (2 marks)

1. _____

2. _____

Jim presented a new guideline for the management of accidental dental trauma. The pathway starts with the pre-operative identification of patients at high risk of dental injury.

d) List four steps that you can take to mitigate the risk of dental injury in a patient with poor dentition planned to undergo lower limb surgery. (4 marks)

1. _____

2. _____

3. _____

4. _____

The meeting ends with an audit presentation by a junior trainee on the incidence of post-operative sore throat.

e) List five factors that increase the risk of a post-operative sore throat. (5 marks)

1. _____

2. _____

3. _____

4. _____

5. _____

Question 10.

Gwendoline is an 87-year-old woman who has been admitted with a fractured neck of femur following a fall at home. She has a background history of hypertension and atrial fibrillation, for which she takes warfarin.

a) According to AAGBI guidelines, within what time period should surgery for hip fracture be performed? (1 mark)

_____

b) List four pre-operative investigations that are indicated based on the clinical history provided above. (4 marks)

1. _____

2. _____

3. _____

4. _____

On further examination, you notice that Gwendoline has an ejection systolic murmur. She is not known to have valvular heart disease.

c) Give two findings from Gwendoline's history and clinical examination that would indicate the need for echocardiography **prior** to anaesthesia. (2 marks)

1. _____

2. _____

d) State three acceptable reasons for delaying surgery for acute hip fracture patients. (3 marks)

1. _____

2. _____

3. _____

Due to her ejection systolic murmur, you opt to perform the procedure under general anaesthesia.

e) Aside from AAGBI standard monitoring and the use of an arterial line, state two other monitoring devices you would consider utilising intra-operatively; give a reason for each. (4 marks)

Monitoring device 1:_____

Clinical reason:_____

Monitoring device 2:_____

Clinical reason:_____

Gwendoline's international normalised ratio is 1.4. You opt to perform a psoas compartment block to supplement her analgesia.

f) Give three potential complications **specific** to this peripheral nerve block. (3 marks)

1. _____

2. _____

3. _____

g) How long after her surgery would you re-instigate Gwendoline's warfarin therapy? (1 mark)

_____

h) If Gwendoline had been a candidate for spinal anaesthesia, what two modifications could you have made to your technique to reduce the risk of intra-operative hypotension? (2 marks)

1. _____

2. _____

Question 11.

a) Describe the molecular structure of adult haemoglobin (Hb). (3 marks)

_____

_____

_____

b) Describe how oxygen (O_2) binds to Hb (2 marks). Explain the term 'cooperative binding'. (1 mark)

O_2 binding to Hb:_____

_____

Cooperative binding:_____

c) List four factors that enhance the binding of O_2 to adult Hb. (4 marks)

1. _____
2. _____
3. _____
4. _____

Hypoxia can be defined as a deficiency in O_2 supply or the inability to utilise O_2.

d) Define the four classes of hypoxia. (4 marks)

_____

_____

_____

_____

e) List the three forms in which carbon dioxide is transported in the blood. (3 marks)

1. _____
2. _____
3. _____

f) Name the enzyme that is essential in facilitating the transport of carbon dioxide. (1 mark)

_____

g) What is the Haldane effect? (1 mark) What is its relevance in the transport of carbon dioxide? (1 mark)

Haldane effect:_____

Relevance:_____

Question 12.

Gillian is a 54-year-old woman listed for vocal cord polypectomy. The surgeons have informed you that the procedure will involve the use of LASER.

a) What does the acronym LASER stand for? (1 mark)

_____

b) State the three characteristic features of laser light. (3 marks)

1. _____
2. _____
3. _____

c) Provide definitions for the following terms implicated in the production of laser light. (3 marks)

Spontaneous emission:_____

Stimulated emission:_____

Population inversion:_____

d) Complete the following table regarding common medical lasers and their applications in clinical practice. (3 marks)

Table 10.12d. **Common medical lasers and their clinical uses**

	Laser medium	Physical state of medium	Application
i		Gas	Cutting, coagulation
ii	Holmium:YAG	Solid	
iii		Gas	Corneal vision correction

e) List two safety features of a laser-resistant endotracheal tube. (2 marks)

1. _____

2. _____

f) List three precautions which are taken to protect theatre staff from injury when using laser light. (3 marks)

1. _____

2. _____

3. _____

g) Despite safety precautions, an airway fire occurs. Give five specific management steps that you would **immediately** take. (5 marks)

1. _____

2. _____

3. _____

4. _____

5. _____

Paper 1 Answers

Question 1 Hydrocephalus

Q	Marking guidance	Mark	Comments
a	• Meningitis • Seizure • Intracranial haemorrhage	Any 2	*Due to tumour recurrence.*
b	**Symptoms:** • Early-morning headache/ headache which is exacerbated by lying flat, coughing, sneezing, bending over, straining • Vomiting • Blurred vision • Diplopia	Any 2	*I.e. the headache is exacerbated by things that cause an acute rise in ICP* *Usually in the absence of nausea* *As a result of papilloedema* *As a result of ocular palsies*
	Signs: • Papilloedema • Seizures • Decreased conscious level • Bradycardia and hypertension • Decerebrate posturing • Fixed dilated pupils • Hemiparesis • Irregular respiration • Death	Any 4	*Papilloedema is a chronic and unpredictable sign.* *This is the Cushing's reflex.*
c	1. Ependymal cells of the choroid plexus (accept either)	1	
	2. Third ventricle through foramina of Monro (need both for 1 mark)	1	*Also known as the interventricular foramina.*
	3. Fourth ventricle through aqueduct of Sylvius (accept canal of Sylvius or cerebral aqueduct) (need both for 1 mark)	1	*Also known as cerebral aqueduct. Long and thin, it is prone to becoming blocked.*
	4. Through foramina of Luschka and Magendie (need both for 1 mark)	1	
	5. Arachnoid granulations	1	*These are located at the superior sagittal sinus.*

(cont.)

Q	Marking guidance	Mark	Comments
d	• Buoyancy	Any 3	*The low specific gravity of CSF reduces the effective weight of the brain from 1.4 kg to just 47 g.*
	• Protection		*Fluid buffer acts as a shock absorber from some forms of mechanical injury.*
	• CSF displacement to compensate for raised intracranial pressure		*Displacement of CSF into the spinal canal is an important compensatory mechanism when ICP is raised.*
	• Provides a constant chemical and ionic environment for neurons		
	• Acid–base regulation for control of respiration		
	• Clearing waste		*CSF is a critical part of the brain's glymphatic system (equivalent of the systemic lymphatic system).*
e	• Set the zero level to the same horizontal level as the foramen of Monro (accept external auditory meatus).	1	*This is equivalent to the external auditory meatus when supine.*
	• Set the drainage level: move the drip chamber to align with the +15 cmH$_2$O marking.	1	
f	• Haemorrhage	Any 2	
	• Infection		*This is the most feared complication: incidence of 5%–20% and high mortality.*
	• Seizure		
	• Sub-optimal placement/ displacement/blockage of catheter		

Suggested reading

H. Krovvidi, G. Flint, A. V. Williams.
   Perioperative management of hydrocephalus.
   BJA Educ 2018; **18**(5): 140–6.

Question 2 Cardiomyopathy

Q	Marking guidance	Mark	Comments
a	Need both elements correct for 1 mark **Dilated:** Stroke volume: low Contractility: low **Hypertrophic:** Cardiac output: low Contractility: high **Restrictive:** Cardiac output: normal or low Stroke volume: low	1 1 1	*Systolic dysfunction is the predominant form of dysfunction that is seen in dilated cardiomyopathy, whereas diastolic dysfunction is the predominant feature of hypertrophic and restrictive cardiomyopathy. Dilated cardiomyopathy occasionally causes a mixed picture of both systolic and diastolic failure.*
b	• Ischaemic • Valvular disease • Post-viral • Peri- and post-partum • Post-chemotherapy • Sickle cell disease • Alcoholism • Hypothyroidism • Muscular dystrophy	Any 3	
c	• Urea and electrolytes (due to ACE inhibitor therapy) • ECG • Transthoracic echocardiography • Full blood count	Any 3	*This patient needs a repeat echo because he has not been to clinic for more than 12 months.*
d	• Five-lead ECG • Invasive arterial blood pressure monitoring • Central venous access • Cardiac output monitoring	Any 3	*The AAGBI recommended standard monitoring includes non-invasive blood pressure monitoring; temperature monitoring; oxygen saturations; inspired and expired carbon dioxide, nitrous oxide and volatile concentrations; three-lead ECG; and peripheral nerve stimulator.*

(cont.)

Q	Marking guidance	Mark	Comments
e	• Avoid tachycardia • Maintain preload/ normovolaemia • Avoid negative inotropy/provide inotropic support • Avoid increases in systemic vascular resistance (SVR) • Maintain afterload/mean arterial pressure (accept avoid reduction in SVR) • Maintain sinus rhythm/rapid treatment of arrhythmias • Intra-operative correction of deranged electrolyte levels	Any 5	*Allowing adequate left ventricular filling in heart failure is critical. Atrial contraction is a key component of ventricular filling; therefore, the aim is to maintain sinus rhythm with a heart rate of 60 beats/min. A low heart rate increases diastolic time, which increases ventricular filling time and allows greater perfusion of the myocardium.* *It is important to avoid precipitous drops in SVR, as a reduction in diastolic blood pressure will impair coronary perfusion.*
f	Advantages: • Reduced risk of tachycardia • Avoidance of increased SVR • Reduction in SVR may increase cardiac output (accept 'reduces sympathetic response to pain' for 1 mark) Disadvantage: • Reduced coronary perfusion with reduction in diastolic BP • Treatment of any hypotension with intravenous fluids increases risk of pulmonary/peripheral oedema	Any 2 Any 1	*Reducing afterload may improve cardiac output; however, hypotension must be avoided due to the risk of myocardial hypoperfusion.* *Remember that SVR and afterload are not the same – afterload relates to ventricular internal fibre load during systole and is a combined effect of SVR alongside the left ventricle chamber pressure, dimensions and wall thickness. Dilated ventricles have an increased afterload.*

Suggested reading

I. R. Ibrahim, V. Sharma. Cardiomyopathy and anaesthesia. *BJA Educ* 2017; **17**(11): 363–9.

Question 3   ICU-Acquired Weakness

Q	Marking guidance	Mark	Comments
a	Clinically detectable weakness in a critically ill patient in whom there is no plausible aetiology other than critical illness	1	
b	Critical illness polyneuropathy (CIP) Critical illness myopathy (CIM) Critical illness neuromyopathy (CINM)	3	*CIM is further subclassified histologically into cachectic myopathy, thick filament myopathy and necrotising myopathy.*
c	• Female sex • Increasing age • Sepsis and septic shock • Multi-organ failure • Drug-induced encephalopathy • Increasing duration of acute illness and immobility • Increasing duration of mechanical ventilation • Requirement for parenteral nutrition • Hypoalbuminaemia • Hyperglycaemia • Use of high-dose steroids • Neuromuscular blocking agents • Vasopressors	Any 6	*The risk of CIM increases with the duration of neuromuscular blockade and corticosteroid use.*
d	• Onset after the acute ICU admission • Generalised, symmetrical weakness • Sparing of the facial muscles/cranial nerves • Difficulties weaning from ventilatory support • Reduced reflexes • Normal conscious level • Medical Research Council power score less than 48	Any 4	*Extra-ocular muscle involvement is rare and suggests an alternative diagnosis.* *Autonomic function is not affected.*

(cont.)

Q	Marking guidance	Mark	Comments
e	Creatine kinase Nerve conduction studies Electromyography Muscle biopsy	4	*Lumbar puncture, erythrocyte sedimentation rate and autoantibodies are often requested to exclude other diagnoses.*
f	45% (accept 40%–50%)	1	
g	68% (accept 60%–70%)	1	

Suggested reading

R. Appleton, J. Kinsella. Intensive care unit-acquired weakness. *Cont Edu Anaesth Crit Care Pain* 2012; **12**(2): 62–6.

Question 4   Caudal Analgesia

Q	Marking guidance	Mark	Comments
a	• Paracetamol • Non-steroidal anti-inflammatory drugs • Opioids (e.g. morphine) • Topical local anaesthetic • Local anaesthetic infiltration • Specific penile block	Any 4	*Topical lidocaine gel, e.g. Instillogel®* *Never use adrenaline-local anaesthetic mix for a penile block!*
b	i = sacrococcygeal membrane (accept sacral hiatus) ii = epidural/caudal space iii = subarachnoid space iv = spinal cord v = dura mater vi = filum terminale	3	1 mark for two correct answers
c	Dural sac ends at S2 (accept S1)	1	*The spinal cord ends at L1/2 in adults and children, and at L3 in an infant*
d	• Intravascular injection/local anaesthetic toxicity • Intrathecal injection/accidental spinal anaesthesia • Hypotension • Block failure (accept subcutaneous injection) • Motor blockade • Urinary retention • Infection/epidural abscess • Epidural haematoma • Accidental needle insertion into rectum/periosteum	Any 4	*The rate of block failure is low at ~2%–5% in experienced hands.*
e	Name = bupivacaine (accept levo-bupivacaine) Concentration = 0.25% Volume = 0.5 mL/kg = 7.5 mL	1 1 1	*For circumcision surgery, a sacro-lumbar block is sufficient, i.e. 0.5 mL/kg. A*

(cont.)

Q	Marking guidance	Mark	Comments
			mid-abdominal block is achieved using 1 mL/kg and a mid-thoracic block by using 1.2 mL/kg of 0.25% bupivacaine.
f	• Fentanyl 1–2 µg/kg = 15–30 µg • Clonidine 1–2 µg/kg = 15–30 µg • Preservative-free ketamine 0.5 mg/kg = 7.5 mg	Any 2	
g	• Physiological (HR, BP, RR) • Behavioural • Self-reporting scales (Piece of Hurt scale/Faces pain scale) • Parent/carer reporting	Any 3	*Assessment of pain in younger patients can be challenging.*

Suggested reading

D. Patel. Epidural analgesia for children. *Cont Edu Anaesth Crit Care Pain* 2006; **6**(2): 63–6.

K. Brand, B. Thorpe. Pain assessment in children. *Anaesth Intensive Care Med* 2016; **17**(6): 270–3.

Question 5 Foetal Well-Being

Q	Marking guidance	Mark	Comments
a	• Baseline (beats/minute) • Baseline variability (beats/minute) • Decelerations	3	*Each feature is described as reassuring, non-reassuring or abnormal.*
b	• Normal • Suspicious • Pathological • Need for urgent intervention	Any 3	*All features reassuring.* *One non-reassuring AND two reassuring features.* *One abnormal feature OR two non-reassuring features.* *Acute bradycardia or prolonged deceleration.*
c	pH: Normal: 7.25 or above Borderline: 7.2–7.25 Abnormal: 7.2 or below Lactate: Normal: 4.1 mmol/L or below Borderline: 4.2 to 4.8 mmol/L Abnormal: 4.9 mmol/L or above	1 1 1 1 1 1	*Be aware that for women with sepsis or significant meconium, foetal blood samples may be falsely reassuring.*
d	Category 1: Immediate threat to the life of the woman or foetus Category 2: Maternal or foetal compromise which is not immediately life threatening Category 3: No maternal or foetal compromise but needs early delivery Category 4: Delivery timed to suit woman or staff	1 1 1 1	*Category 1: target time from decision to delivery is <30 min.* *Category 2: target time from decision to delivery is <75 min.* *Delivery should always be carried out with an urgency appropriate to the risk of the baby and the safety of the mother, regardless of classification.*

(cont.)

Q	Marking guidance	Mark	Comments
e	• Malpresentation • Multiple pregnancy – first twin is not cephalic	Any 4	*Women with breech babies should be offered external cephalic version (ECV) at 36 weeks. If unsuccessful, a planned caesarean section (CS) should be offered.*
	• Placenta praevia • Abnormally adherent placenta • Transmissible disease: HIV, genital HSV		*HIV infection does not mandate a CS. Where viral loads are >400 copies/mL or no anti-retrovirals are being taken, CS is considered.* *CS does not reduce the transmission of hepatitis B or C.*
	• Cephalopelvic disproportion • Previous caesarean section • Maternal request • Maternal conditions: diabetes, cardiovascular disease • Previous traumatic delivery		

Suggested reading

G. Jayasooriya, V. Djapardy. Intrapartum assessment of fetal well-being. *BJA Educ* 2017; **17**(12): 406–11.

National Institute for Health and Care Excellence Clinical Guideline 190: Intrapartum care for healthy women and babies. 2014. www.nice.org.uk/guidance/cg190. (Accessed 1 September 2018).

Question 6 Rib Fractures

Q	Marking guidance	Mark	Comments
a	• Atelectasis • Hypoxaemia/shunt • Pneumothorax • Haemothorax • Pneumonia • Respiratory failure/need for intubation • Hypercapnoea/need for non-invasive ventilation	Any 5	*A greater number of fractured ribs, and especially a flail segment, indicates a greater likelihood of underlying pulmonary contusion.*
b	• Humidified oxygen • Nebulised saline • Chest physiotherapy	Any 2	*Humidification helps to loosen secretions and improves sputum clearance.*
c	• Non-steroidal anti-inflammatory drugs (NSAIDs) • Oral morphine as required • Antiemetics	Any 2	*This patient has a rib fracture score of 5 (three unilateral ribs fractured, plus two for ages 61–70). He should be offered an NSAID and enteral morphine before moving to parenteral morphine.*
d	**Regional anaesthetic technique 1.** Thoracic epidural Advantage: excellent analgesia Disadvantage: technically difficult to insert; risk of dural puncture/spinal cord injury; hypotension **Regional anaesthetic technique 2.** Paravertebral block Advantage: fewer side effects, e.g. hypotension; can cover up to five levels with one paravertebral catheter Disadvantage: risk of epidural spread, pneumothorax	 1 1 Any 1 1 Any 1 Any 1	Not acceptable: interpleural block or intercostal block – higher risk of local anaesthetic toxicity *Epidural analgesia has traditionally been used to manage more complex rib fractures. However, many trauma patients are multiply injured, and adequate positioning, hypotension and coagulopathy remain prime concerns. Alternative*

(cont.)

Q	Marking guidance	Mark	Comments
	<u>Regional anaesthetic technique 3.</u> Serratus plane block Advantage: superficial block; performed with patient supine; can be inserted in anticoagulated patients Disadvantage: pneumothorax; vascular puncture	1 Any 1 Any 1	*regional techniques have* *fewer side effects and offer* *near-equivalent analgesia.*

e	Fixation recommended if
	• ≥5 fractured ribs with a flail
	  segment, particularly if the
	  patient requires invasive or
	  non-invasive ventilation
	• Symptomatic non-union
	• Severely displaced ribs found
	  during a thoracotomy for
	  another reason
		Any 2	*Rib fixation has recently*
			seen a resurgence of
			interest, with a number of
			trials demonstrating benefit
			in the most severely injured
			trauma patients. Benefits
			include reduced pneumonia
			rates, shorter critical care
			stays and fewer ventilated
			days.

Suggested reading

L. May, C. Hillermann, S. Patil. Rib fracture management. *BJA Educ* 2016; **16**(1): 26–32.

M. de Moya, R. Nirula, W. Biffl. Rib fixation: who, what, when? *Trauma Surg Acute Care Open* 2017; **2**(1): e000059. http://tsaco.bmj.com/content/2/1/e000059. (Accessed 18 August 2018).

Question 7 Bone Cement Implantation Syndrome

Q	Marking guidance	Mark	Comments
a	Grade 1: <94% O_2 saturations >20% reduction in systolic BP No change in conscious level Grade 2: <88% O_2 saturations >40% reduction in systolic BP Loss of consciousness	3 3	*BCIS occurs around the time of cementation, prosthesis insertion, reduction of the joint or (rarely) deflation of the tourniquet in patients undergoing cemented bone surgery.*
b	Cardiovascular collapse/ cardiopulmonary resuscitation	1	
c	• ASA III–IV • Pulmonary hypertension • Significant cardiac/pulmonary disease • Osteoporosis • Male	Any 3	
d	Hypoxia: • Increase in pulmonary artery pressure (accept increased pulmonary vascular resistance) • $\dot{V}/\dot{Q}$ mismatch Hypotension: • Dilatation of the right ventricle • Shifting of interventricular septum, which reduces left ventricular compliance/filling and cardiac output	1 1 1 1	*Various theories for the development of BCIS exist, e.g. systemic release of cement polymer, cement monomer, air or medullary fat during cementation may initiate histamine release and complement activation.*
e	• 100% O_2 • Volume resuscitation • Consider drugs to achieve positive inotropy (β_1-agonists) • Pulmonary vasodilators • Vasopressors • Invasive monitoring (arterial line, central line, cardiac output monitoring)	Any 4	*Treatment is supportive and should be aggressive. BCIS is a reversible, time-limited phenomenon: pulmonary artery pressures usually normalise within 24 hours.*

(cont.)

Q	Marking guidance	Mark	Comments
	• Secure the airway		
f	• Lavage of femoral canal before cementing • Depressurising the intramedullary canal • Brushing and drying of the intramedullary canal pre-cementation • Using a bone-vacuum cementing technique • Retrograde insertion of cement • Using low-viscosity cement	Any 2	*Venting the bone by drilling holes in the cortical bone creates a pressure-releasing vent for cementation, which reduces the incidence of air embolus. Unfortunately, drilling also increases the risk of femoral fracture.*

Suggested reading

J. Donaldson, H. E. Thomson, N. J. Harper, N. W. Kenny. Bone cement implantation syndrome. *Br J Anaesth* 2009; **102**(1): 12–22.

G. Khanna, J. Cernovsky. Bone cement and the implications for anaesthesia. *Cont Edu Anaesth Crit Care Pain* 2012; **12**(4): 213–6.

D. So, C. Yu. Bone Cement Implantation Syndrome. World Federation of Societies of Anaesthesiologists' Anaesthesia Tutorial of the Week 351. 2017. www.wfsahq.org/compo nents/com_virtual_library/media/e952a87 e99551930e9ca80f8a885f813-374-psu.pdf. (Accessed 21 October 2018).

Question 8   Hyperthyroidism

Q	Marking guidance	Mark	Comments
a	• Iodide (I⁻) uptake	4	I^- is actively transported into the thyroid follicular cells through a Na^+/I^- co-transporter. This process is stimulated by thyroid stimulating hormone (TSH).
	• I⁻ oxidation		I^- is oxidised to the more reactive I_2 by hydrogen peroxide. This process is stimulated by TSH.
	• I₂ reaction with tyrosine		Tyrosine in the surrounding thyroglobulin reacts with I_2, resulting in mono-iodotyrosine (MIT) or di-iodotyrosine (DIT).
	• Oxidative coupling		Two iodinated tyrosine molecules couple. Coupling of two DIT molecules produces T_4, whilst coupling of MIT to DIT produces T_3. Coupling is stimulated by TSH.
b	• Agitation/restlessness • Anxiety • Fine tremor • Weight loss despite increased appetite • Tachycardia/palpitations/atrial fibrillation • Intolerance to heat • Sweating • Diarrhoea • Palmar erythema • Proximal myopathy • Hair loss (especially outer third of eyebrow) • Oligomenorrhoea • High output cardiac failure	Any 6	Not acceptable: Graves' ophthalmopathy symptoms/signs or pretibial myxoedema, as these are specific to Graves' disease and not hyperthyroidism. Many of the clinical features of hyperthyroidism can be accounted for by a TSH-induced upregulation of β_1-receptors and an increase in basal metabolic rate. β-blockers may be helpful to control tachycardia, palpitations and tremor.

(cont.)

Q	Marking guidance	Mark	Comments
c	• Graves' disease • Multinodular thyroid • Thyroiditis: Hashimoto's thyroiditis and subacute (de Quervain's) thyroiditis • Toxic thyroid adenoma • Pituitary adenoma causing TSH hypersecretion	Any 2	*Graves' disease is the most common cause of hyperthyroidism in the United Kingdom. The pathophysiology is autoimmune: autoantibodies (thyroid stimulating immunoglobulin, TSI) are raised that stimulate the thyroid gland to release thyroid hormones. The autoantibodies of Graves' disease also result in eye disease (exophthalmos) and pretibial myxoedema.*
d	A low thyroid stimulating hormone (TSH) concentration (<0.4 mU/L) A high free T_4 concentration > 25 pmol/L	1 1	*The hypothalamic-pituitary-thyroid axis is normally controlled by negative feedback.*
e	Antithyroid drugs: • Propylthiouracil • Carbimazole Radioiodine (I-131)	Any 2	*Propylthiouracil works by preventing the conversion of T_4 to the active thyroid hormone T_3.* *Carbimazole prevents the production of T_4 by inhibiting the iodination of thyroglobulin by thyroperoxidase.* *I-131 is actively taken up into thyroid tissue, where it causes local destruction.*
f	• Haemorrhage causing airway obstruction • Tracheomalacia	Any 4	*A tense neck swelling may result in stridor and dyspnoea.* *Tracheomalacia – partial tracheal collapse resulting in dynamic airway obstruction.*

(cont.)

Q	Marking guidance	Mark	Comments
	• Recurrent laryngeal nerve palsy		*Intra-operative electromyography may be used to minimise this complication.*
	• Laryngeal oedema		
	• Hypocalcaemia, which may cause laryngospasm		*Acute hypocalcaemia is due to inadvertent excision of the parathyroid glands, which lie posterior to the four poles of the thyroid gland.*

Suggested reading

S. Malhotra, V. Sodhi. Anaesthesia for thyroid and parathyroid surgery. *Cont Edu Anaesth Crit Care Pain* 2007; **7**(2): 55–8.

L. Adams, S. Davies. Anaesthesia for thyroid surgery. World Federation of Societies of Anaesthesiologists' Anaesthesia Tutorial of the Week 162. 2009. www.aagbi .org/sites/default/files/162-Anaesthesia-for -thyroid-surgery.pdf. (Accessed 18 August 2018).

Question 9   Pre-operative Anaemia

Q	Marking guidance	Mark	Comments
a	• Chronic haemorrhage • B$_{12}$ deficiency • Folate deficiency • Iron deficiency • Alcohol excess • Hypothyroidism • Anaemia of chronic disease • Haemolytic anaemia • Thalassaemias • Sickle cell disease	Any 4	Not acceptable: acute haemorrhage, which is not a cause of *chronic* anaemia.
b	Microcytic iron deficiency anaemia	1	
c	• Tiredness/lethargy • Palpitations/tachycardia • Dizziness/syncope • Dyspnoea • Pallor/pale conjunctiva • Flow murmurs • Signs of high output heart failure	Any 4	
d	Intravenous iron (e.g. ferric carboxymaltose) Not acceptable: oral iron, e.g. ferrous fumerate	1	*The patient has severe anaemia and likely ongoing gastrointestinal blood loss – oral iron is likely to be ineffective.*
e	• Cell salvage • Intravenous tranexamic acid • Meticulous surgical technique/ consultant surgeon • Use of intra-operative topical haemostatic agents • Minimise the use of surgical drains • Use of central neuraxial blockade • Maintenance of balanced physiology • Point-of-care coagulation testing	Any 8	*NB a leucocyte depletion filter should be used, as it reduces the risk of re-introducing cancer cells.* *E.g. microfibrillar collagen, recombinant thrombin.* *I.e. avoiding hypothermia, acidosis, hypocalcaemia.* *TEG® or ROTEM®*

Q	Marking guidance	Mark	Comments
	• Reducing the frequency and volume of intra-operative and post-operative blood sampling • Prescribe further intravenous iron post-operatively • Accept lower transfusion triggers Not acceptable: minimally invasive surgical techniques. Whilst these are associated with reduced blood loss, this lady is already listed for laparoscopic surgery.		*E.g. use of paediatric blood bottles* *NICE recommends a transfusion trigger of 70 g/L, or 80 g/L in patients with underlying cardiovascular disease.*
f	• Increased risk of cancer recurrence • Lower survival rates • Increased risk of surgical site infection • Increased risk of post-operative pulmonary complications	Any 2	

Suggested reading

S. V. Thakrar, B. Clevenger, S. Mallett. Patient blood management and perioperative anaemia. *BJA Educ* 2017; **17**(1): 28–34.

Question 10   Electroconvulsive Therapy

Q	Marking guidance	Mark	Comments
a	Fluoxetine: Class: selective serotonin reuptake inhibitor	1	*Patients presenting for ECT have, by definition, severe depression. Many patients take a combination of many psychoactive drugs, some of which have a significant bearing on anaesthetic management.*
	Interaction: tramadol or pethidine may precipitate serotonin syndrome	1	
	Amitriptyline: Class: tricyclic antidepressant	1	
	Interaction: potentiation of the effect of indirectly acting sympathomimetics	1	
	Phenelzine: Class: monoamine oxidase inhibitor	1	
	Interaction: profound pressor response following administration of directly and indirectly acting sympathomimetics	1	
b	Unilateral electrode position over non-dominant hemisphere	1	
	Advantage: reduces memory loss	1	
	Bilateral electrode position	1	
	Advantage: more rapid clinical effects	1	
c	• Initial parasympathetic nervous system activation	1	
	• Causes bradycardia, hypotension or asystole	1	
	• Followed by sympathetic nervous system activation	1	
	• Causes hypertension, increased myocardial oxygen consumption	1	
d	• Recent (3 months) myocardial infarction	Any 4	
	• Recent (3 months) stroke		
	• Presence of raised intracranial pressure		
	• Uncontrolled cardiac failure		
	• Deep vein thrombosis (not anticoagulated)		
	• Untreated cerebral aneurysm		

(cont.)

Q	Marking guidance	Mark	Comments
	• Unstable major fracture • Severe osteoporosis • Phaeochromocytoma • Retinal detachment • Glaucoma		
e	• Neuromuscular blockade (usually suxamethonium, dose 0.5 mg/kg) to reduce the intensity of the convulsions	1	*The Bolam test originated from a case in which an anaesthetist did not use muscle relaxant during ECT*
	• A bite block is used to protect the teeth, tongue and lips	1	*and the patient suffered an acetabular fracture.*

Suggested reading

T. Peck, A. Wong, E. Norman. Anaesthetic implications of psychoactive drugs. *Cont Edu Anaesth Crit Care Pain* 2010; **10**(6): 177–81.

V. Uppal, J. Dourish, A. Macfarlane. Anaesthesia for electroconvulsive therapy. *Cont Edu Anaesth Crit Care Pain* 2010; **10**(6): 192–6.

Question 11 Anaphylaxis

Q	Marking guidance	Mark	Comments
a	• Hypotension • Tachycardia or bradycardia • Low end-tidal carbon dioxide • Bronchospasm/high airway pressures • Hypoxaemia/low oxygen saturations • Urticaria/rash/flushing • Angioedema • Cardiac arrest	Any 4	*Hypotension is the most common sign of anaphylaxis.*
b	• Antibiotics • Muscle relaxants • Surgical cleaning solutions (chlorhexidine) • Patent blue dye (used in some breast surgery)	1 1 1 1	*Penicillins and teicoplanin were most commonly reported in NAP6.*
c	1:10,000 anaesthetics (0.01%)	1	*According to NAP6*
d	• 100% oxygen • Stop administering all potentially causative agents • Adrenaline 50 µg (0.5 mL of 1:10,000 solution) intravenously/0.5 mg intramuscularly • Intravenous fluid bolus	4	*Measures to treat persistent bronchospasm (e.g. intravenous/endotracheal salbutamol, magnesium), and chlorphenamine/ hydrocortisone are not accepted, as these are not* **initial** *management.*
e	• Type 1 hypersensitivity reaction • Initial sensitisation/IgE produced • IgE coats mast cells • On subsequent exposure, mast cells degranulate • Substances released include histamine	1 1 1 1 1	*Substances released from mast cells include histamine, heparin, leukotrienes, prostaglandin D2 and platelet activating factor.*
f	Test: mast cell tryptase Timings: as early in the resuscitation as possible, at 1–2 hours and at 24+ hours (three samples)	1 1	*Following anaphylaxis, the peak in mast cell tryptase occurs between 1 and 2 hours.*

Suggested reading

A. T. D. Mills, P. J. A. Sice, S. M. Ford. Anaesthesia-related anaphylaxis: investigation and follow-up. *Cont Edu Anaesth Crit Care Pain* 2014; 14(2): 57–62.

Anaesthesia, surgery and life-threatening allergic reactions. Report and findings of the Royal College of Anaesthetists Sixth National Audit Project: Perioperative anaphylaxis. www.niaa.org.uk/NAP6Report?newsid=1914#pt. (Accessed 8 August 2018).

Association of Anaesthetists of Great Britain and Ireland. Suspected anaphylactic reactions associated with anaesthesia. 2009. www.aagbi.org/sites/default/files/anaphylaxis_2009_0.pdf. (Accessed 8 August 2018).

Question 12   Abdominal Aortic Aneurysm

Q	Marking guidance	Mark	Comments
a	• Less surgically invasive • Potentially shorter duration of surgery for simpler aneurysms • Avoids short-term complications of laparotomy • Avoids long-term complications of laparotomy • Reduced haemodynamic and metabolic stress • Decreased morbidity and mortality • Large blood transfusion unlikely • Early ambulation possible • Decreased length of stay	Any 6	 *E.g. ileus, pneumonia* *E.g. incisional hernia* *With a corresponding reduction in the risk of perioperative myocardial infarction.*
b	• Age > 70 years • Diabetes mellitus • Cardiac failure • Pre-operative eGFR < 60 mL/min (CKD stage 3a and above) • Perioperative dehydration • Angiotensin-converting enzyme (ACE) inhibitor/angiotensin II receptor blocker therapy • Perioperative administration of aminoglycosides/diuretics • Repeat exposure to intravenous contrast within 7 days • Complex EVAR (fenestrated/chimney/branched graft)	Any 6	
c	• Limit intravenous contrast dose • Prevent intra-operative dehydration/pre-procedure intravenous fluid • *N*-acetyl cysteine (NAC)	Any 4	 *Supported by a number of meta-analyses.*

Q	Marking guidance	Mark	Comments
	• Sodium bicarbonate		*The evidence supporting bicarbonate therapy is less robust than NAC.*
	• Omit nephrotoxic drugs		*E.g. ACE inhibitors, non-steroidal anti-inflammatory drugs.*
	• Maintenance of an adequate mean arterial pressure (MAP)		*The optimum target MAP is not clear but is probably within 10% of pre-operative blood pressure and is certainly ≥ 65 mmHg.*
d	<u>Indications for CRT:</u> • New York Heart Association class III or IV symptoms • Either QRS duration ≥ 150 ms with left bundle branch block or mechanical dyssynchrony on echocardiogram • Left ventricular ejection fraction ≤ 35%	Any 2	
	<u>Perioperative implications:</u> • Pre-operative device check • Deactivate defibrillator/anti-tachycardia functions in anaesthetic room • Apply anterior–posterior defibrillation pads • Continue biventricular pacing intra-operatively	Any 4	*Depending on the device, this may be done by applying a magnet to the skin overlying the device.* *Continuing biventricular pacing maintains ventricular synchrony, which improves cardiac output whilst under general anaesthesia.*
	• Avoid unipolar diathermy • Avoid suxamethonium • Reinstate defibrillator function immediately post-operatively		*Fasciculations may be misinterpreted by the device.*

Suggested reading

V. Nataraj, A. J. Mortimer. Endovascular abdominal aortic aneurysm repair. *Cont Edu Anaesth Crit Care Pain* 2004; **4**(3): 91–4.

V. Kasipandian, A. C. Pitchel. Complex endovascular aortic aneurysm repair. *Cont Edu Anaesth Crit Care Pain* 2012; **12**(6): 312–6.

Paper 2 Answers

Question 1 Prone Position

Q	Marking guidance	Mark	Comments
a	Motor evoked potentials (MEPs) Somatosensory evoked potentials (SSEPs)	2	
b	Volatile anaesthetics and nitrous oxide depress the amplitude of SSEPs and MEPs	1	*A normal dose of muscle relaxant at induction of anaesthesia is acceptable. Traditionally, a low muscle relaxant infusion titrated to 1–2 twitches is then used, but now, more commonly, a remifentanil infusion is used to facilitate intra-operative ventilation.*
	Muscle relaxants (full paralysis) make MEPs useless	1	
c	• Pillows	Any 4	
	• Chest/pelvic bolsters		
	• Allen/Jackson table		*A frame in which the patient is supported by a chest block and iliac crest/ thigh supports.*
	• Montreal mattress		*A foam mattress with a cut-out for the abdomen.*
	• Wilson frame		*The Wilson frame is used for lumbar surgery: a winding mechanism increases the radius of curvature, thus reducing lumbar lordosis.*
	• Knee–chest position		

(cont.)

Q	Marking guidance	Mark	Comments
d	• Brachial plexus injury.	Any 4	*If head is turned to right/ left, or shoulders abducted > 90° angle.*
	• Post-operative visual loss		*Most commonly due to ischaemic optic neuropathy and central retinal artery occlusion.*
	• Peripheral nerve injury		
	• Spinal cord injury		*Rolling with unstable fractures, or with over-extension or over-flexion of the cervical spine.*
	• Increased intracranial pressure		*Due to obstruction of cerebral venous drainage (head rotated/not neutral).*
	• Ischaemic stroke/spinal cord ischaemia as a result of hypotension		
e	• Reduced cardiac output/ hypotension due to inferior vena cava compression leading to reduced preload	Any 6	*With good prone positioning (in the absence of abdominal compression), functional residual capacity actually increases. This is the physiological basis of prone positioning of patients with acute respiratory distress syndrome.*
	• Intra-operative venous bleeding due to raised epidural venous pressure		
	• Lower limb venous thrombosis due to inferior vena cava compression		
	• Decrease in respiratory compliance		
	• Decreased left ventricular compliance due to raised intrathoracic pressure		
	• Acute kidney injury		
	• Increased intragastric pressure		
	• Acute liver injury/metabolic acidosis		

(cont.)

Q	Marking guidance	Mark	Comments
f	Alert: Ventilator signals a 'low-pressure' alarm/reservoir bag empties/surgical admission of guilt	1	*The priority in this situation is to establish that the patient can be ventilated. A decision can*
	Manage airway: Insert a laryngeal mask airway Bag–mask ventilation	Any 1	*then be made either to continue with an LMA in place or to exchange for an endotracheal tube, e.g. by using the LMA as a conduit for fibre-optic intubation.*

Suggested reading

B. Fiex, J. Sturgess. Anaesthesia in the prone position. *Cont Edu Anaesth Crit Care Pain* 2014; **14**(6): 291–7.

H. Edgcombe, K. Carter, S. Yarrow. Anaesthesia in the prone position. *Br J Anaesth* 2008; **100**(2): 165–83.

Question 2 Post-cardiac Transplant

Q	Marking guidance	Mark	Comments
a	• Resting heart rate 90–100 beats/min • Baroreceptor reflex lost – hypotension does not trigger tachycardia • Laryngoscopy does not cause tachycardia • Pneumoperitoneum does not cause reflex bradycardia • Changes in heart rate are no longer an indicator of depth of anaesthesia • Cardiac output is dependent on adequate preload • Cardiac dysrhythmias are more common	Any 4	*The transplanted heart has no autonomic innervation. Neither a tachycardia nor a bradycardia can be mounted in response to usual physiological triggers.*
b	<u>Vagolytics:</u> • Atropine and glycopyrrolate have no effect on heart rate <u>Inotropic/chronotropic drugs:</u> • Increased sensitivity to adrenaline and noradrenaline • No effect of indirectly acting sympathomimetics, e.g. ephedrine <u>Antiarrhythmics:</u> • Marked sensitivity to adenosine – dose reduction needed • Digoxin is ineffective for the treatment of atrial fibrillation <u>Other:</u> • No reflex tachycardia with glyceryl trinitrate • No bradycardia with neostigmine or suxamethonium	Any 4	
c	• Recent echocardiogram to assess graft function • ECG • CMV status • Electrolytes	Any 2	

(cont.)

Q	Marking guidance	Mark	Comments
d	• Awake arterial line • Central venous line • Aim for normovolaemia prior to induction of anaesthesia • Maintain coronary perfusion pressure/correct hypotension • Scrupulous asepsis for lines and urinary catheter • Availability of chronotropic/inotropic drugs, and external pacemaker • Immunosuppression therapy should be continued perioperatively	Any 4	*The transplanted heart cannot reflexly respond to sudden changes in systemic vascular resistance (SVR). Therefore, it is important to maintain normovolaemia, instigate beat-to-beat blood pressure monitoring, and have the means to rapidly correct anaesthetic-induced decreases in SVR (i.e. a central line).*
e	Mycophenolate and tacrolimus should both be given in the morning before surgery. Patient first on the list/timing to reduce risk of missed doses Liaison with transplant team regarding immunosuppression Both drugs have parenteral preparation in the event of impaired gastrointestinal absorption Drug levels – drug concentrations may be increased or decreased through drug–drug interactions	Any 3	*It is imperative that immunosuppression is continued throughout the perioperative period.*

(cont.)

Q	Marking guidance	Mark	Comments
f	• Chronic allograft vasculopathy (CAV, accelerated coronary atherosclerosis) • Malignancy, mainly skin cancers • Renal failure • Diabetes mellitus • Opportunistic infections, e.g. *Pneumocystis jirovecii* • Hypertension	Any 3	*CAV is thought to take place through a chronic rejection mechanism.* *Renal failure and diabetes are side effects of the immunosuppressive agents.* *New hypertension may occur secondary to anti-rejection drugs.*

Suggested reading

N. J. Morgan-Hughes, G. Hood. Anaesthesia for a patient with a cardiac transplant. *BJA CEPD Reviews* 2002; **2**(3): 74–8.

Question 3 Brainstem Death and Organ Donation

Q	Marking guidance	Mark	Comments
a	NHS blood and transplant	1	
b	The irreversible loss of the capacity for consciousness, combined with the irreversible loss of the capacity to breathe	1	*As defined by the Academy of Medical Royal Colleges.*
c	• Irreversible structural brain damage of known aetiology causing unresponsive coma	1	*All four preconditions must be met for the diagnosis of brainstem death to be valid.*
	• The absence of any depressant drugs or neuromuscular blocking agents	1	
	• Normothermia (i.e. core temperature > 34°C)	1	
	• No significant metabolic disturbances (i.e. normal blood sugar and electrolytes)	1	
d	At the end of the first set of brainstem death tests	1	*Two complete sets of tests need to be performed but the recorded time of death is at the end of the first set.*

(cont.)

Q	Marking guidance	Mark	Comments
e	One mark for a correct physiological derangement, and 1 mark for a correct corresponding reason.	8	
	• Hypothermia → hypothalamic damage leading to reduced metabolic rate, vasodilatation and heat loss		*Heat-generating metabolic processes are reduced.*
	• Hypotension → vasoplegia; hypovolaemia; reduced coronary blood flow leading to myocardial dysfunction		
	• Diabetes insipidus → posterior pituitary damage as a result of raised intracranial pressure		
	• Disseminated intravascular coagulation (DIC) → tissue factor release leading to widespread coagulation		*Coagulopathy is common following isolated head injury (occurs in up to one-third of patients). Following brainstem death, tissue thromboplastin is released from the necrotic brain, which contributes to DIC.*
	• Arrhythmias → 'catecholamine storm' leading to myocardial damage		*Raised intracranial pressure causes an increase in sympathetic nervous system activity, as the brain attempts to maintain cerebral perfusion pressure. After the catecholamine storm, there is a loss of sympathetic tone, leading to peripheral vasodilatation and hypotension. If untreated, this leads to organ hypoperfusion, including the heart, and may contribute to rapid donor loss.*

(cont.)

Q	Marking guidance	Mark	Comments
	• Pulmonary oedema → acute blood volume diversion, pulmonary capillary damage		
f	• CO_2 diffuses across blood–brain barrier into the cerebrospinal fluid • Fall in CSF pH stimulates the central chemoreceptors • Peripheral chemoreceptors in the carotid body and aortic arch detect changes in arterial P_aCO_2 and pH • Peripheral chemoreceptors send afferent impulses via the glossopharyngeal and vagus nerves • Central chemoreceptors play a greater role than peripheral chemoreceptors in the control of ventilation, but the response to peripheral chemoreceptors is more rapid • The medullary respiratory centre is stimulated to increase the rate and depth of ventilation.	Any 4	*The peripheral chemoreceptors are responsible for around 20% of the ventilatory response to hypercapnoea, with the central chemoreceptors responsible for the remainder. The response from the peripheral chemoreceptors is rapid, within the order of 1–3 seconds.* *The carotid bodies (but not the aortic bodies or central chemoreceptors) also respond to acidaemia (plasma pH < 7.35).*
g	0.5 kPa (accept 0.5–0.65 kPa)	1	

Suggested reading

J. Oram, P. Murphy. Diagnosis of death. *Cont Edu Anaesth Crit Care Pain* 2011; **11**(3): 77–81.

D. McKeown, R. Bonser, J. Kellum. Management of the heartbeating brain-dead organ donor. *Br J Anaesth* 2012; **108**(Suppl. 1): 96–107.

Question 4   Child Protection

Q	Marking guidance	Mark	Comments
a	Physical	1	
	Sexual	1	
	Emotional	1	
	Neglect	1	
b	<u>Child-related factors:</u>	Any 6	
	• Chronic disability/illness		
	• Prematurity/low birth weight		
	• Unplanned/unwanted child		
	• Learning difficulties/behavioural problems		
	<u>Parental factors:</u>		
	• Step parent		
	• Teenage parent		
	• Substance abuse		
	• Parent abused as a child		
	• Disabled parent		
	• Mental health problems		
	<u>Family factors:</u>		
	• Single-parent family		
	• Domestic violence		
	<u>Social factors:</u>		
	• Unemployment		
	• Poverty		
	• Isolation		
c	<u>Neurological:</u>	Any 6	*The differential diagnosis for the unconscious infant is wide, and includes pathophysiology other than non-accidental injury.*
	• Seizure/febrile seizure/post-ictal state		
	• Central nervous system infection		
	• Intracerebral haemorrhage/ diffuse axonal injury		
	• Hydrocephalus		
	<u>Infective:</u>		
	• Sepsis		
	<u>Metabolic:</u>		
	• Hypo/hyperglycaemia		
	• Hepatic encephalopathy		
	<u>Poisoning:</u>		
	• Drugs, alcohol		

Q	Marking guidance	Mark	Comments
d	• Consultant anaesthetist • Person with level 3 child safeguarding competencies • On-call paediatrician	Any 1	*The GMC emphasises the importance of sharing information with other agencies, even if that means breaking confidentiality, if the child is at significant risk of harm.*
e	• Level 1 = administrative and clerical staff with paediatric patient contact, e.g. theatre receptionist	1	One mark for type **plus** example
	• Level 2 = all clinical staff with paediatric patient contact, e.g. scrub nurse, anaesthetist	1	
	• Level 3 = clinical staff with extensive and regular contact with paediatric patients, and have a level of responsibility in assessing, planning and evaluating patient needs when safeguarding concerns are raised. E.g. lead paediatric anaesthetist, tertiary paediatric anaesthetist.	1	

Suggested reading

K. Melarkonde, K. Wilkinson. Child protection issues and the anaesthetist. *Cont Edu Anaesth Crit Care Pain* 2012; **12**(3): 123–7.

Question 5 Pre-eclampsia

Q	Marking guidance	Mark	Comments
a	• Sustained increase in BP • BP ≥ 140/90 mmHg • After 20 weeks gestation • Previously normotensive patient	4	
b	• Chronic kidney disease • Autoimmune disease such as systemic lupus erythematosus or antiphospholipid syndrome • Pre-existing diabetes mellitus • BMI > 35 kg/m²	Any 3	*Other risk factors include:* *Age > 40 years* *Nulliparity/multiparity* *Family history of pre-eclampsia Interpregnancy gap of >10 years*
c	• Severe headache • Visual problems such as blurring or flashing before the eyes • Subcostal pain/liver tenderness • Vomiting • Sudden swelling of the face, hands or feet	Any 4	*Severe pre-eclampsia is diagnosed when there is proteinuria with severe hypertension (≥160/100 mmHg) or when there is hypertension (≥140/90 mmHg) plus one of these clinical features.*
d	• Urinary protein : creatinine ratio > 30 • 24-hour urine protein collection > 300 mg	Any 1	*Proteinuria signifies the endothelial damage characteristic of pre-eclampsia.*
e	• Raised transaminases (ALT/AST > 70 IU) • Raised creatinine • Thrombocytopenia (platelets < 100 × 10⁹/L)	3	*The combination of haemolysis, elevated liver enzymes and low platelets (HELLP) often results in significant maternal morbidity and, occasionally, mortality.*
f	• Labetalol at a dose of 50 mg (accept 20–50 mg) • Hydralazine at a dose of 5 mg (accept 5–10 mg) • Nifedipine at a dose of 10 mg (accept 5–10 mg)	Any 2	*BP control is essential for the prevention of intracerebral haemorrhage in pre-eclampsia.*

Q	Marking guidance	Mark	Comments
g	Drug: magnesium sulphate Dose: 4 g slow intravenous injection Infusion: 1 g/hour for 24 hours	3	*Magnesium is the treatment of choice for eclampsia and is used in severe pre-eclampsia to reduce the risk of progression to eclampsia.*

Suggested reading

D. Leslie, R. E. Collis. Hypertension in pregnancy. *BJA Educ* 2016; **16**(1): 33–7.

National Institute for Health and Care Excellence. Hypertension in pregnancy: the management of hypertensive disorders during pregnancy CG107. 2010. www.nice.org.uk/guidance/cg107. (Accessed 20 October 2018).

Question 6 Trigeminal Neuralgia

Q	Marking guidance	Mark	Comments
a	• Paroxysmal attacks of facial pain lasting a few seconds to 2 min • Paroxysms often triggered by benign stimuli: smiling, brushing teeth, shaving • Character of pain: intense, sharp, superficial or stabbing • Affecting one or more divisions of the trigeminal nerve • Unilateral facial pain	Any 3	
b	• Cluster headache • Dental pain from dental abscess • Temporomandibular joint disorder • Other neuralgias, e.g. post-herpetic neuralgia • Sinusitis • Tumours, e.g. acoustic neuroma, meningioma	Any 4	
c	• Compression by blood vessels • Multiple sclerosis • Compression by tumours	3	
d	Carbamazepine	1	*The first-line agent, with a number needed to treat of 1.8.*

(cont.)

Q	Marking guidance	Mark	Comments
e	Surgical option 1:		
	Neurolysis of trigeminal nerve branch using alcohol injection or laser	1	
	Advantage: less invasive	1	
	Disadvantage: short-term pain relief (~6 months to 1 year); dysaesthesias	1	
	Surgical option 2:		
	Ablation of trigeminal ganglion	1	*Using radiofrequency*
	Advantage: longer-term pain relief (few years)	1	*ablation, chemical (phenol, alcohol, glycerol) or*
	Disadvantage: high incidence of anaesthesia and dysaesthesias in the nerve distribution; anaesthesia dolorosa; cardiac arrhythmias; aseptic meningitis; temporary diplopia	1	*mechanical (balloon compression) techniques.*
	Surgical option 3:		
	Microvascular decompression	1	*The trigeminal nerve root is*
	Advantage: high initial success rate (80%–90%)	1	*physically separated from compressing vessel, and*
	Disadvantage: craniotomy required (mortality 0.5%); aseptic meningitis; hearing loss; anaesthesia in trigeminal nerve distribution; CSF leak; intracranial haematoma	1	*kept separate using a small Teflon spacer.*

Suggested reading

C. K. Vasappa, S. Kapur, H. Krovvidi. Trigeminal neuralgia. *BJA Educ* 2016; **16**(10): 353–6.

Question 7 Rheumatoid Arthritis

Q	Marking guidance	Mark	Comments
a	• Proximal interphalangeal (PIP) • Metacarpophalangeal (MCP) • Wrists • Shoulders • Neck • Elbows • Ankles	Any 2	*The distal interphalangeal joints are generally spared.*
b	• Atlanto-axial subluxation • Narrowed glottis due to amyloidosis and rheumatoid nodules • Temporomandibular joint involvement causing limited mouth opening	3	*Acute subluxation may result in spinal cord compression and/or vertebral artery compression, leading to quadriparesis or sudden death.*
c	Respiratory: • Fibrosing alveolitis → restrictive lung deficit • Costochondral disease → reduced chest wall compliance • Pleural effusions → reduced lung volumes Cardiovascular: • Pericardial effusions → cardiac tamponade, reduced cardiac output • Granulomatous disease → cardiac conduction defects • Myocarditis → left ventricular failure, reduced cardiac output • Peripheral vasculitis/Raynaud's phenomenon → difficulty reading peripheral oxygen saturations	Any 10	1 mark for each systemic feature **plus** anaesthetic relevance. *Approximately 50% of rheumatoid arthritis patients have extra-articular disease.*

(cont.)

Q	Marking guidance	Mark	Comments
	Haematological: • Anaemia of chronic disease → patient blood management • Iron deficiency anaemia due to non-steroidal anti-inflammatory use → pre-operative iron therapy **Renal:** • Renal amyloidosis → renal impairment, reduced drug clearance **Neurological:** • Autonomic neuropathy → impaired reflex response to intra-operative hypotension • Peripheral neuropathy → care with positioning, risk of perioperative nerve injury • Kerato-conjunctivitis → risk of corneal abrasions – care when taping eyelids closed **Skin:** • Thin skin/easy bruising due to steroid treatment → positioning difficulty		
d	• Hypertension → intra-operative cardiovascular instability • Obesity → manual handling • Thin skin → care with positioning and removing dressings • Hypokalaemia → cardiac arrhythmias • Adrenal suppression → perioperative steroid replacement • Diabetes mellitus → impaired wound healing • Immunosuppression → increased risk of post-operative infection	Any 3	1 mark for each feature **plus** perioperative relevance. *Perioperative steroid replacement is required for patients taking > 10 mg prednisolone. For this surgery, the patient's normal prednisolone should be given, plus 25 mg hydrocortisone at induction, plus 100 mg hydrocortisone in divided doses for 2–3 days.*

(cont.)

Q	Marking guidance	Mark	Comments
e	• Etanercept	Any 2	*Binds tumour necrosis factor (TNF)*
	• Infliximab		*Anti-TNF antibody*
	• Adalimumab		*Anti-TNF antibody*
	• Anakinra		*Blocks activity of interleukin-1*

Suggested reading

F. N. Fombon, J. P. Thompson. Anaesthesia for the adult patient with rheumatoid arthritis. *Cont Edu Anaesth Crit Care Pain* 2006; 6(6): 235–9.

Question 8 Malignant Hyperthermia

Q	Marking guidance	Mark	Comments
a	Autosomal dominant	1	
b	• Volatile anaesthetic agents (accept: isoflurane/sevoflurane/ desflurane/halothane) • Suxamethonium	1 1	
c	Central core disease	1	*An inherited disorder characterised by peripheral muscle weakness; the only disease in which there is a confirmed association with MH.*
d	• Action potential arrives at terminal bouton → • ACh release in NMJ → • AChR at motor end plate → • Cations enter ion channel → • Cell membrane depolarises → • Spread into muscle along T-tubules → • DHPR conformational change → • Ryanodine receptor (RyR) triggers • SR to release Ca^{2+} into cell → • Excitation–contraction coupling	Any 6	ACh = acetylcholine AChR = ACh receptor NMJ = neuromuscular junction DHPR = dihydropyridine receptor SR = sarcoplasmic reticulum
e	• Ryanodine (RyR) receptor mutation • Release large amounts of Ca^{2+} from the SR into the cell	1 1	
f	• Hypermetabolism (tachycardia, hypercarbia/increased end-tidal CO_2, lactic acidosis, tachypnoea, hypoxaemia, hyperthermia) • Rhabdomyolysis (hyperkalaemia/cardiac arrhythmias, acidosis, myoglobinuria/acute renal failure, disseminated intravascular coagulation) • Muscle rigidity	Up to 2 Up to 2 1	

(cont.)

Q	Marking guidance	Mark	Comments
	• Masseter spasm	1	
	• Hypertension	1	
g	• Change circuits • Flush with 100% O_2 at maximal flows for 20–30 min • Use of charcoal filters	Any 2	*The aim being complete removal of volatile agent from the anaesthetic apparatus.*
h	• Genetic testing • Muscle biopsy/caffeine–halothane contracture test	1 1	*Genetic testing may only confirm a diagnosis of MH if an abnormal gene is identified; it cannot exclude MH susceptibility.*

Suggested reading

P. K. Gupta, P. M. Hopkins. Diagnosis and management of malignant hyperthermia. *BJA Educ* 2017; **17**(7): 249–54.

Question 9   Needlestick Injury

Q	Marking guidance	Mark	Comments
a	1 in 3 for hepatitis B (33%) (accept 20%–40%)	1	*The high risk of hepatitis B transmission is why all healthcare workers are inoculated against hepatitis B.*
	1 in 30 for hepatitis C (3.3%) (accept 2%–4%)	1	
	1 in 300 for HIV (0.33%) (accept 0.2%–0.4%)	1	
b	• Deep injuries	Any 4	
	• Hollow-bore needle		*Due to the higher volume of blood inoculated.*
	• Blood visible on the needle		
	• Needle which has been in a vein or artery of an HIV-positive source patient		
	• Advanced disease or high viral load		
c	Make the injury bleed	1	
	Wash under the tap	1	
d	Hepatitis B inoculation	1	
	Hepatitis C immunoglobulin	1	
	HIV post-exposure prophylaxis	1	
e	Commence within an hour, certainly within 24 hours	1	
	Duration of course: 28 days	1	
f	Combination drug: Truvada	1	*According to the most recent UK guidelines.*
	Constituent drugs:		
	• Emtricitabine/'nucleoside reverse transcriptase inhibitor (NRTI)' class	1	
	• Tenofovir/'nucleotide reverse transcriptase inhibitor (NRTI)' class	1	
g	• Prolonged headaches	Any 3	*The question asks for common side effects. Rare side effects include lactic acidosis and liver dysfunction.*
	• Abdominal pain		
	• Nausea/vomiting		
	• Diarrhoea		
	• Weight loss		
	• Decreased bone density		

Suggested reading

P. Ward, A. Hartle. UK healthcare workers infected with blood-borne viruses: guidance on risk, transmission, surveillance, and management. *Cont Edu Anaesth Crit Care Pain* 2015; 15(2): 103–8.

Question 10   Post-operative Nausea and Vomiting

Q	Marking guidance	Mark	Comments
a	Within 48 hours of surgery	1	
b	• Prolonged admission • Electrolyte derangement • Dehydration • Suture dehiscence • Aspiration injury • Oesophageal rupture • Failure of enteral medication • Emotional distress/unpleasant symptom	Any 4	*Surveys have consistently found that many patients find PONV more distressing than post-operative pain.*
c	• Female gender • History of PONV • Non-smoker • Perioperative opioid use	4	*Motion sickness is NOT included in the simplified Apfel score.*
d	60%	1	*PONV risk per Apfel score is: 0 = 10% risk, 1 = 20% risk, 2 = 40% risk, 3 = 60% risk, 4 = 80% risk*
e	<u>Ondansetron:</u> Dose: 4 mg Activity: serotonin 5-HT$_3$ receptor antagonist Timing: induction	2	*A new 5-HT$_3$ receptor antagonist, Palonosetron, has no effect on QT$_c$ interval and has a longer duration.*
	<u>Droperidol:</u> Dose: 0.625–1.25 mg Activity: dopamine D$_2$ receptor antagonist Timing: end of surgery	3	
	<u>Dexamethasone:</u> 4–8 mg Activity: unknown Timing: induction	2	

(cont.)

Q	Marking guidance	Mark	Comments
	Aprepitant: Dose: 40 mg Activity: neurokinin-1 receptor antagonist Timing: pre-induction	2	*NK-1 receptor antagonists are a promising new class of antiemetics originally developed for chemotherapy. Aprepitant is not associated with QT_c prolongation or sedative effects, but its high cost limits its use.*
	Metoclopramide: Dose: 25–50 mg Activity: dopamine D_2 receptor antagonist Timing: induction	1	*Metoclopramide does not have any effect on PONV at a dose of 10 mg.*

Suggested reading

S. Pierre, R. Whelan. Nausea and vomiting after surgery. *Cont Edu Anaesth Crit Care Pain* 2012; **13**(1): 28–32.

Question 11 Total Intravenous Anaesthesia

Q	Marking guidance	Mark	Comments
a	• Malignant hyperthermia (MH) risk • Long QT syndrome (QT$_c$ ≥ 500 ms)	Any 6	*The volatile anaesthetics are all triggers for MH. Whilst volatile anaesthetics prolong the QT interval, they do not tend to promote torsades de pointes.*
	• History of severe post-operative nausea and vomiting • 'Tubeless' ENT/thoracic surgery • Surgery requiring neurophysiological monitoring		*Volatile agents interfere with motor evoked potentials.*
	• Anaesthesia/transfer in non-theatre environments • Patients with anticipated difficult airway		*Volatile anaesthesia may be only intermittently delivered during a difficult intubation.*
	• Day surgery		*TIVA has very good recovery characteristics.*
	• Neurosurgery		*TIVA offers a theoretical advantage over volatile anaesthetics in the reduction of cerebral blood flow and thus decreased intracranial volume.*
	• Cancer surgery		*An increasing body of evidence suggests improved cancer survival with TIVA techniques. This is probably because volatile anaesthetics inhibit natural killer cell activity.*
b	Marsh Schnider	2	.

(cont.)

Q	Marking guidance	Mark	Comments
c	• C_1 = Central compartment • C_2 = Vessel-rich peripheral compartment • C_3 = Vessel-poor peripheral compartment • Drug is injected into the central compartment • Drug is eliminated from the central compartment • Drug moves from C_1 to C_2, and C_1 to C_3 until equilibrium is reached • Transfer between compartments is governed by rate constants	Any 5	*The pharmacokinetic compartments do not strictly relate to anatomical structures. In the three-compartment model, C_1 can be thought of as plasma, with C_2 as highly perfused structures (e.g. brain, heart and muscles), and C_3 as lipid-rich structures (e.g. adipose tissue).*
d	• High infusion pressure alarm • Low infusion pressure alarm • End of infusion warning • Disengagement of driver warning • Low battery/disconnection from mains electricity • Displays the selected drug and concentration on-screen • User confirms the syringe type and size • Syringe driver service record alert	Any 5	*Alerts the user to a possible occlusion.* *Alerts the user to a possible disconnection.* *Prompts the anaesthetist to draw up a new syringe.* *To reduce the risk of wrong-drug infusion.* *To ensure the correct rate of infusion.* *Aids regular syringe driver service.*
e	Zero-order kinetics: a constant amount of a drug is eliminated per unit time, i.e. the elimination rate is no longer proportional to drug concentration. Example: phenytoin; heparin; ethanol; aspirin/salicylates; theophylline; warfarin.	1 1	*This is due to saturation of the elimination process (usually an enzyme).*

Suggested reading

D. J. Chambers. Principles of intravenous infusion. *Anaesth Intensiv Care Med* 2019; **20**(1): 61–4.

Z. Al-Rifai, D. Mulvey. Principles of total intravenous anaesthesia: practical aspects of using total intravenous anaesthesia. *BJA Educ* 2016; **16**(8): 276–80.

Z. Al-Rifai, D. Mulvey. Principles of total intravenous anaesthesia: basic pharmacokinetics and model descriptions. *BJA Educ* 2016; **16**(3): 92–7.

Question 12 Penetrating Eye Injury

Q	Marking guidance	Mark	Comments
a	i = cornea ii = iris iii = lens iv = ciliary body v = fovea vi = retina vii = choroid viii = sclera	4	No half marks, 1 mark for two correct answers.
b	• Produced by ciliary body • In posterior chamber • Drains between iris and anterior lens • Through pupil into anterior chamber • Exits eye through trabecular network/canal of Schlemm	Any 4	
c	Ketamine Suxamethonium	1 1	
d	• Fentanyl (3–5 µg/kg) • Alfentanil (20 mcg/kg) • Lignocaine (1.5 mg/kg) • Remifentanil TCI (C_{et} 3–5 ng/mL)	Any 2	NB – the dose of opioids needed to attenuate the sympathetic response to laryngoscopy is higher than those typically used for intra-operative analgesia.
e	• Head-up tilt • Avoid hypercarbia (P_aCO_2 4.5–5.5 kPa) • Intravenous mannitol (0.5 g/kg) • Intravenous acetazolamide (500 mg) • Reduce/avoid obstruction to venous blood flow • Ensure adequate depth of anaesthesia/analgesia	Any 4	Many of these strategies used to reduce intraocular pressure mirror those used to reduce intracranial pressure.

(cont.)

Q	Marking guidance	Mark	Comments
f	• Insert orogastric tube to suction stomach contents • Extubation with background opioid (further opioid bolus or infusion) • Deep extubation in spontaneously breathing patient • Exchange endotracheal tube for laryngeal mask airway • Administer antiemetic drugs • Prescribe post-operative antiemetic drugs	Any 4	*The aim here is to reduce coughing, bucking and retching on emergence and in the immediate post-operative period.*

Suggested reading

I. James. Anaesthesia for paediatric eye surgery. *Cont Edu Anaesth Crit Care Pain* 2008; **8**(1): 5–10.

Paper 3 Answers

Question 1 Spinal Cord Injury

Q	Marking guidance	Mark	Comments
a	1. Shoulder abduction = C5 2. Elbow flexion = C6 (accept C5) 3. Elbow extension = C7 4. Finger abduction = T1	4	*Mnemonic: 'C5/6 – pick up sticks, C7/8 keep it straight'*
b	Hypotension due to decreased systemic vascular resistance	1	*Due to interruption of sympathetic neurons*
	Bradycardia as a result of unopposed vagal tone	1	*Due to interruption of sympathetic cardioacceleratory neurons*
c	• Rapid shallow breathing • High cervical cord injury • Vital capacity < 15 mL/kg; serial vital capacity measurement worsening trend • Hypercapnoea/P_aCO_2 > 6.0 kPa • Poor cough • Patient fatigue	Any 4	*Respiratory failure is very common in cervical spinal cord injury. It is always better to perform a semi-elective as opposed to emergent intubation, as the latter is more likely to lead to neurological injury through neck manipulation or hypoxaemia.*
d	• Manual in-line stabilisation • Rapid sequence induction Not acceptable: avoidance of suxamethonium, as extra-junctional acetylcholine receptors do not develop for 48 hours.	2	*Gastric emptying is reduced in high spinal cord injury.*

Q	Marking guidance	Mark	Comments
e	• Lung-protective ventilation/ 6–8 mL/kg tidal volume	Any 8	
	• Chest physiotherapy		
	• Tracheostomy		*Improved patient comfort, allows cessation of sedation.*
	• Vasopressors		*The mean arterial blood pressure target in spinal cord injury remains controversial.*
	• Catheterisation		*Prevents bladder overdistension, which may precipitate reflex bradycardia.*
	• Maintenance of spinal alignment/ log rolling		*Thought to prevent secondary cord injury.*
	• Spinal surgical referral/early surgical fixation		*Early surgical fixation aids mobilisation, reducing the risk of developing pressure sores.*
	• Thromboprophylaxis		
	• Gut protection (prophylactic H_2-receptor antagonist or proton pump inhibitor)		*Unopposed vagal activity increases gastric acid secretion and peptic ulceration.*
	• Glycaemic control		*The stress response to trauma results in hyperglycaemia.*
	• Bowel care/laxatives		*Unopposed vagal input may result in paralytic ileus.*
	• Enteral nutrition		
	• Prevent pressure sores, e.g. pressure-relieving mattress, early surgical fixation		
	• Normothermia		
	• Full secondary survey		

Suggested reading

S. Bonner, C. Smith. Initial management of acute spinal cord injury. *Cont Edu Anaesth Crit Care Pain* 2013; **13**(6): 224–31.

M. Denton, J. McKinlay. Cervical cord injury and critical care. *Cont Edu Anaesth Crit Care Pain* 2009; **9**(3): 82–6.

Question 2   Ischaemic Heart Disease

Q	Marking guidance	Mark	Comments
a	• History of congestive cardiac failure	1	*Lee's Revised Risk Score of 0 = 0.4% risk of major intra-operative cardiac event, score 1 = 0.9% risk, score 2 = 6.6% risk, score ≥ 3 = 11% risk.*
	• History of cerebrovascular disease	1	
	• Diabetes mellitus **requiring insulin**	1	
	• High-risk surgical procedure	1	
	• Creatinine >176 µmol/L (accept 170–180 µmol/L)	1	
b	6.6% (accept 6–7%)	1	*Insiya scores two: one for 'ischaemic heart disease' and one for 'high-risk surgery'*
c	Oxygen supply:	Any 3	
	• Diastolic time (not acceptable: heart rate)		
	• Coronary perfusion pressure (accept diastolic blood pressure)		
	• Arterial oxygen content		
	• Haemoglobin concentration		
	• Coronary artery diameter		
	Oxygen demand:	Any 3	
	• Heart rate		
	• Ventricular wall tension		
	• Afterload (accept systemic vascular resistance)		
	• Contractility		
d	Pharmacodynamic rationale: Reduces left ventricular end-diastolic pressure (accept reduced wall tension)	1	*By reducing wall tension, GTN reduces myocardial oxygen demand and increases sub-endocardial O_2 supply through increased coronary blood flow.*
	Dose: 10–200 µg/min	1	
e	Cardiogenic shock (accept cardiac/left ventricular failure)	1	

(cont.)

Q	Marking guidance	Mark	Comments
f	Drug class: Specific phospho-diesterase III inhibitor	1	*Milrinone and enoximone are other examples of the so-called inodilators.*
	Mechanism of action: Prevents degradation of cyclic adenosine monophosphate (accept increases intracellular cAMP, accept increases intracellular calcium movement)	1	
g	• Intra-aortic balloon pump • Urgent revascularisation • Left ventricular assist device (accept LVAD)	1 1 1	*In a non-cardiac centre, these options may not be readily available!*

Suggested reading

K. Webster. Acute Coronary Syndrome. World Federation of Societies of Anaesthesiologists' Anaesthesia Tutorial of the Week 210. 2011. www.aagbi.org/sites/default/files/210-Acute-Coronary-Sydnromes.pdf. (Accessed 6 September 2018).

G. Minto, B. Biccard. Assessment of the high-risk perioperative patient. *Cont Edu Anaesth Crit Care Pain* 2013; **14**(1): 12–7.

H. S. Koh, J. Rogers. Anaesthesia for patients with cardiac disease undergoing non-cardiac surgery. World Federation of Societies of Anaesthesiologists' Updates in Anaesthesia. www.e-safe-anaesthesia.org/e_library/05/An aesthesia_for_patients_with_cardiac_disea se_undergoing_non.pdf. (Accessed 22 August 2018).

Question 3   Propofol-Related Infusion Syndrome

Q	Marking guidance	Mark	Comments
a	• Refractory bradycardia leading to asystole • Other cardiac arrhythmia, e.g. supraventricular tachycardia	Any 7	*PRIS was originally described by Bray in the paediatric population in 1998 and has subsequently been reported in adult patients.*
	• Metabolic acidaemia		*Base deficit greater than (more negative than) –10 mmol/L, due to lactate acidosis.*
	• Rhabdomyolysis		*Due to myocyte necrosis → myoglobinuria/acute renal failure.*
	• Hyperkalaemia (plasma K^+ > 5.5 mmol/L) • Lipaemic plasma		*Due to hypertriglyceridaemia.*
	• Enlarged/fatty liver • Progressive myocardial collapse/ cardiac failure		
b	4 mg/kg/h	1	*Whilst the quoted 'safe' dose is 4 mg/kg/h, fatal cases of PRIS have been reported after infusion doses as low as 1.9 mg/kg/h. Genetic factors may play a role in the susceptibility of a patient to PRIS.*
c	• Severe head injuries • Sepsis • Pancreatitis • High endogenous or exogenous catecholamine or glucocorticoid levels • Low carbohydrate supply leading to increased lipolysis during times of starvation, e.g. burns or trauma • Inborn errors of fatty acid oxidation • Paediatric population	Any 4	*Children are more prone to the development of PRIS due to low glycogen storage and high dependence on fat metabolism.*

(cont.)

Q	Marking guidance	Mark	Comments
d	• Acidaemia (pH < 7.35) • Raised lactate (>2 mmol/L) • Elevated creatine kinase, with no other obvious cause • Myoglobinuria • Hyperkalaemia (>5.5 mmol/L) • Hypertriglyceridaemia (>1.9 mmol/L) • Raised serum creatinine	Any 3	
e	• Cessation of propofol infusion, use of alternative sedation • Inotropic or vasopressor support • Cardiac pacing for refractory bradycardia • Haemodialysis to resolve acidaemia/renal failure • Adequate carbohydrate administration to suppress lipolysis, minimising lipid load (e.g. avoiding TPN) • Extracorporeal membrane oxygenation (ECMO) has been used for combined respiratory and cardiovascular support	4	*There is no specific treatment for PRIS, just supportive measures to counteract its consequences.*
f	Literature estimates range from 4% to 18%	1	

Suggested reading

N. Loh, P. Nair. Propofol infusion syndrome. *Cont Edu Anaesth Crit Care Pain* 2013; **13**(6): 200–2.

Question 4 Down's Syndrome

Q	Marking guidance	Mark	Comments
a	Trisomy 21: the presence of a third copy of chromosome 21	1	*95% of patients with Down's syndrome have this genetic abnormality. The remainder have a chromosomal translocation (4%) or mosaic trisomy 21 (1%).*
b	Prenatal: • Amniocentesis • Chorionic villous sampling Postnatal: • Genetic testing (chromosomal karyotype) using blood sample Not acceptable: screening tests (e.g. nuchal translucency)	Any 2	*Prenatal diagnostic testing carries a small risk of miscarriage, and is offered when screening tests predict a high risk of Down's syndrome.*
c	• Brachycephaly • Flat occiput • Flat nasal bridge • Brushfield spots in iris • Epicanthic folds • Upwardly slanting palpebral fissures • Small mouth • Macroglossia • Small ears • Single transverse palmar (Simian) crease • Obesity • Short stature • Short neck • 'Sandal gap' between first and second toes	Any 6	

(cont.)

Q	Marking guidance	Mark	Comments
d	• Congenital heart disease (CHD): atrial, atrioventricular and ventricular septal defects, patent ductus arteriosus, tetralogy of Fallot (accept up to two CHD answers) • Subglottic stenosis • Duodenal atresia • Hirschsprung's disease • Pyloric stenosis • Meckel's diverticulum • Imperforate anus	Any 4	*Around 50% of babies born with Down's syndrome have a congenital cardiac defect. Mitral valve prolapse is a common finding in adults with Down's syndrome. Found in up to 8% of patients.* *Eight percent of Down's infants have duodenal atresia.*
e	Acute myeloid leukaemia (AML)	1	*AML is 500 times more common in Down's syndrome, whilst acute lymphoblastic leukaemia is 20 times more common. It is thought that leukaemogenic genes may be located on chromosome 21.*
f	Atlantoaxial instability (AAI) Cervical spondylosis	1 1	*Asymptomatic AAI is found in between 10% and 20% of Down's syndrome children. Two percent of children have symptomatic AAI.* *Increasing incidence with age: ~70% by age 40.*
g	• Craniofacial abnormalities • Obstructive sleep apnoea (OSA) • Small mouth • Macroglossia • Micrognathia • Short neck • Adenotonsillar hypertrophy	Any 4	*OSA is very common, and is due to both craniofacial changes and obesity.*

Suggested reading

J. E. Allt, C. J. Howell. Down's syndrome. *BJA CEPD Rev* 2003; **3**(3): 83–6.

K. Melarkode. Anaesthesia for children with Down's syndrome. World Federation of Societies of Anaesthesiologists' Anaesthesia Tutorial of the Week 139. 2009. www.aagbi.org/sites/default/files/139-Anaesthesia-for-children-with-downs-syndrome.pdf. (Accessed 11 August 2018).

Question 5   Amniotic Fluid Embolism

Q	Marking guidance	Mark	Comments
a	Obstetric: • Eclampsia • Uterine rupture • Placental abruption • Peripartum cardiomyopathy • Uterine inversion	Any 3	*When faced with maternal collapse, ensure all potential causes are considered. AFE is a diagnosis of exclusion.*
	Non-obstetric causes: • Sepsis • Pulmonary embolism • Air/fat embolism • Pulmonary oedema • Heart failure • Myocardial infarction • Anaphylaxis • High spinal • Local anaesthetic toxicity • Intracranial haemorrhage • Drug reaction	Any 3	*The reported incidence of AFE ranges from 1:8000 to 1:80,000, and it accounts for 4.7% of direct maternal deaths in the UK. AFE occurs most commonly during labour, but can occur during Caesarean section and following delivery. Neonatal mortality is high (70%) and neurological injury is common in survivors.*
b	• Foetal compromise • Cardiac arrest • Cardiac rhythm abnormalities • Hypotension • Coagulopathy • Haemorrhage • Seizure • Dyspnoea/cyanosis	Any 5	*The UKOSS criteria are based on acute maternal collapse with one or more of the stated features, in the absence of a more likely diagnosis.*
c	Mechanical/embolic Immune/humoural	1 1	*Both theories hypothesise exposure of the maternal circulation to amniotic fluid or foetal antigens.*

(cont.)

Q	Marking guidance	Mark	Comments
d	Left ventricular failure/pulmonary oedema	1	*Phase 1 (lasts up to 30 min): pulmonary artery vasospasm, pulmonary hypertension, right ventricular failure, hypoxaemia and hypotension. Phase 2: left ventricular failure and pulmonary oedema, DIC.*
	Disseminated intravascular coagulation (DIC)/coagulopathy	1	
e	• Call for help • Left lateral tilt or manual displacement • Airway management • Cardiopulmonary resuscitation • Deliver baby	5	*Management in AFE is supportive. Multi-disciplinary management and early senior help is key.* *Think about delivery of the baby early. Expect and plan for massive haemorrhage in maternal survivors. Complete UKOSS AFE register.*

Suggested reading

Y. Metodiev, P. Ramasamy, D. Tuffnell. Amniotic fluid embolism. *BJA Educ* 2018; **18**(8): 234–8.

Royal College of Obstetrics and Gynaecology. Maternal collapse in pregnancy and puerperium: Green-top guideline No. 56. 2011. www.rcog.org.uk/globalassets/documents/guidelines/gtg_56.pdf. (Accessed 10 August 2018).

Question 6 Low Back Pain

Q	Marking guidance	Mark	Comments
a	i = Vertebral body ii = Pedicle iii = Lamina iv = Spinous process v = Superior articular process (accept facet joint) vi = Central spinal canal	3	No half marks, 1 mark for two correct answers
b	<u>History</u> • Age of onset < 16 or > 50 years old • History of significant trauma • Thoracic pain • Bladder or bowel dysfunction • Constitutional symptoms: unexplained weight loss, fever, night sweats • Nocturnal back pain • Previous history of malignancy • Immunosuppression (e.g. long-standing steroid use, HIV infection) • Intravenous drug abuse • Presence of other medical illnesses/recent significant infection • Gait disturbance <u>Clinical signs</u> • Perianal/perineal sensory loss (saddle anaesthesia) or paraesthesias • Reduced anal tone • Hip or knee weakness • Point tenderness over the vertebral body • Severe or progressive neurological deficit in legs • Pyrexia	Any 5 Any 5	

(cont.)

Q	Marking guidance	Mark	Comments
c	Discogenic pain	1	*Accounts for 40% of mechanical back pain, difficult to distinguish from other causes of lower back pain.*
	Sacroiliac joint pain	1	*Accounts for 20% of mechanical back pain. Pain arising from this joint is rarely present above the transverse process of L5. Stressing the joint may reproduce the patient's pain.*
	Lumbar facet joint pain	1	*Accounts for 10%–15% of mechanical back pain in young patients, up to 40% in elderly. Characterised by pain that is worsened by rotation and extension, radiation into the leg, tenderness over the joints and paravertebral muscle spasm.*
d	• A belief that back pain is harmful or potentially severely disabling • Fear avoidance behaviour and reduced activity levels • An expectation that passive, rather than active, treatment will be beneficial • A tendency to depression, low morale, and social withdrawal • Social or financial problems	Any 4	*These psychosocial factors are often referred to as 'yellow flags', whilst the symptoms and signs of serious spinal pathology are commonly called 'red flags'.*

Suggested reading

M. A. Jackson, K. H. Simpson. Chronic back pain. *Cont Edu Anaesth Crit Care Pain* 2006; **6**(4): 152–5.

Question 7 Accidental Awareness under General Anaesthesia

Q	Marking guidance	Mark	Comments
a	Explicit awareness: conscious recollection of events, either spontaneously or as a result of direct questioning	2	*Intra-operative explicit awareness may be with or without pain.*
	Implicit awareness: implicit memories exist without conscious recall, but they can alter behaviour after the event	2	
b	• Neuromuscular blockade • Caesarean section • Thiopentone use • Rapid sequence induction • Total intravenous anaesthesia • Female patients • Early middle-age patients • Out-of-hours operating • Junior anaesthetists • Previous episode of AAGA	Any 6	Not acceptable: induction and emergence – these are the most common phases of anaesthesia to experience awareness, but are not risk factors. *These were the factors highlighted in the Royal College of Anaesthetists Fifth National Audit Project as being 'over-represented'. Caesarean section carries the highest risk, at 1:670.*
c	• Involve consultant anaesthetist • See the patient accompanied by a nurse/midwife • Establish the exact nature of the awareness, i.e. explicit vs implicit, pain sensation experienced? • Always believe the patient and empathise • Explain the nature of the anaesthetic and how the awareness could have occurred • Invite questions from the patient, and offer follow-up – return at a later date, counselling, follow-up obstetric anaesthetic clinic	Any 3	*It is important to establish whether this is truly a case of AAGA, or whether this was awareness of awake extubation. AAGA may cause significant psychological harm, such as anxiety/fear of future surgery and anaesthesia, sleep disturbances and flashbacks, nightmares and post-traumatic stress disorder.*

(cont.)

Q	Marking guidance	Mark	Comments
	• Inform general practitioner • Document all events carefully • Follow hospital critical incident reporting procedures		
d	• Clinical signs/observations • Isolated forearm technique • Lower oesophageal contractility • End-tidal volatile concentration • Frontalis electromyogram (EMG) • Electroencephalogram (EEG)-based (maximum 2 marks): pure EEG, Bispectral index (BIS), Narcotrend, M-Entropy. • Evoked potentials: auditory, motor, sensory	Any 4	*The clinical signs of AAGA may be pharmacologically masked. Hypertension and tachycardia may be masked by antihypertensives and β-blockers. Anticholinergics may prevent lachrymation and cause mydriasis.*
e	Wakefulness: fine wave/β-wave activity	1	*Processed EEG, for example BIS, analyse the raw EEG for these wave patterns, and display a number between 0 and 100 corresponding to the depth of anaesthesia. Between 40 and 60 is considered a surgical plane of anaesthesia.*
	Surgical anaesthesia: spindle waves/ α-waves, θ (theta)/δ (delta) waves	1	
	Excessive anaesthesia: burst suppression	1	

Suggested reading

N. Goddard, D. Smith. Unintended awareness and monitoring of depth of anaesthesia. *Cont Edu Anaesth Crit Care Pain* 2013; **13**(6): 213–7.

J. J. Pandit, J. Andrade, D.G. Bogod, et al. 5th National Audit Project (NAP5) on accidental awareness during general anaesthesia: summary of main findings and risk factors. *Br J Anaesth* 2014; **113**(4): 549–59.

Question 8 Tubeless Surgery

Q	Marking guidance	Mark	Comments
a	• Tobacco: smoked or chewed	Any 4	*Tobacco use is the single greatest risk factor in the development of oropharyngeal cancer.*
	• Alcohol • Human papillomavirus (HPV) infection • Male sex • Age > 55 years • Poor oral hygiene		*The number of oropharyngeal cancers linked to HPV has increased dramatically – the cause is unclear.*
b	• Microlaryngoscopy tube and intermittent positive pressure ventilation • Supraglottic jet ventilation • Subglottic jet ventilation • Trans-tracheal jet ventilation	Any 2	
c	Total intravenous anaesthesia	1	*It is not possible to deliver volatile anaesthetic agents using HFNOT.*
d	HFNOT delivers: • Warmed (33°–43°C) • Humidified gas (95%–100% humidity) • At greater flow rate up to 60 L/min (must state flow rate for the mark)	Any 2	*Traditional nasal cannulae deliver cold, dry oxygen. Patient discomfort generally limits the flow rate to ≤ 4 L/min.*
e	• Intubation and difficult airway • Maintenance of oxygenation at extubation • Post-operative hypoxaemia • Procedural oxygenation: dental procedures, awake fibre-optic intubation, bronchoscopy (Not acceptable: critical care applications)	Any 2	*HFNOT significantly extends the apnoeic period.*

(cont.)

Q	Marking guidance	Mark	Comments
f	Warmed humified gas: • Improved clearance of secretions • Decreased atelectasis High gas flow: • Washout of anatomical dead space • Allows F_iO_2 close to 100% to be delivered Positive end-expiratory pressure (PEEP): • Low level of PEEP delivered whether mouth open or closed • Increased functional residual capacity • Alveolar recruitment	Any 5	*Dry, cold gas impairs ciliary function.* *Patients require a lower minute ventilation to achieve the same alveolar ventilation.* *A much higher F_iO_2 can be delivered due to reduced entrainment of air.* *The evidence base for HFNOT remains small: HFNOT has been shown to be non-inferior to non-invasive ventilation in certain critical care patients.*
g	• Type 2 respiratory failure • Unconscious patients • Uncooperative patients • Basal skull fracture • Epistaxis • Facial injury • Laser surgery • Airway/nasal obstruction	Any 4	*This could potentially result in pneumocephalus.* *Most HFNOT equipment can only deliver 100% oxygen, which risks airway fire.*

Suggested reading

B. H. Millett, V. Athanassoglou, A. Patel. High flow nasal oxygen therapy in adult anaesthesia. *Trends Anaesth Crit Care* 2018; **18**: 29–33.

N. Ashraf-Kashani, R. Kumar. High-flow nasal oxygen therapy. *BJA Educ* 2017; **17**(2): 63–7.

A. Ahmed-Nusrath. Anaesthesia for head and neck cancer surgery. *BJA Educ* 2017; **17**(12): 383–9.

Question 9 Phaeochromocytoma

Q	Marking guidance	Mark	Comments
a	Phaeochromocytoma	1	
b	• Epinephrine/adrenaline • Norepinephrine/noradrenaline • Dopamine • Chromogranin A • Opioid peptides • Vasoactive intestinal peptide (VIP) • Adrenocorticotropin (ACTH) • Calcitonin • Somatostatin • Neuropeptide Y	Any 4	*Although phaeochromocytomas usually predominantly secrete noradrenaline or adrenaline, they are capable of secreting many other peptides.*
c	• Headache • Palpitations • Sweating • Anxiety • Lethargy • Nausea • Weight loss • Hyperglycaemia • Tremor	Any 4	*The classic triad associated with phaeochromocytoma is paroxysms of headache, palpitations and sweating, with or without hypertension.*
d	Metanephrine Normetanephrine Not acceptable: vanillylmandelic acid (VMA), the concentration of which is measured in a 24-hour **urine** collection	Any 1	*The result of the metabolism of adrenaline by COMT.* *The result of the metabolism of noradrenaline by COMT.*
e	• Arterial pressure control: phenoxybenzamine or doxazocin • Heart rate/arrhythmia control: selective β_1-blockers (e.g. atenolol, bisoprolol, metoprolol)	1 1	*Phenoxybenzamine = non-selective, non-competitive, long-acting α-blocker* *Doxazocin = competitive, selective α_1-blocker*

(cont.)

Q	Marking guidance	Mark	Comments
	• Investigation of myocardial function: ECG, echocardiogram	1	
	• Management of hyperglycaemia: e.g. metformin, gliclazide, insulin	1	
f	• Magnesium sulphate • Phentolamine • Sodium nitroprusside (SNP)/ glyceryl trinitrate (GTN) • Nicardipine • Esmolol Not acceptable: remifentanil – whilst it is effective in blunting haemodynamic response to laryngoscopy or pain, it is ineffective in treating hypertensive crises associated with tumour manipulation	Any 4	*Magnesium sulphate is usually given prophylactically – it inhibits adrenal catecholamine release and reduces α-adrenergic receptor sensitivity to catecholamines.* *Phentolamine = reversible non-selective α-blocker, 1–2 mg bolus.* *SNP and GTN are both nitric oxide donors, administered by infusion.* *Nicardipine = dihydropyridine Ca^{2+} channel antagonist, administered by infusion.* *Esmolol = selective β_1-blocker, administered by infusion.*
g	• Multiple endocrine neoplasia (types 2A and 2B) • Von Hippel–Lindau disease • Neurofibromatosis • Succinate dehydrogenase enzyme deficiency	Any 2	

Suggested reading

D. Connor, S. Boumphrey. Perioperative care of phaeochromocytoma. *BJA Educ* 2016; **16**(5): 153–8.

Question 10   Awake Fibre-optic Intubation

Q	Marking guidance	Mark	Comments
a	• A clinical situation in which an anaesthetist experiences difficulty with facemask ventilation, supraglottic device ventilation, tracheal intubation or all three • >2 attempts at intubation using direct laryngoscopy (same or different blade) • Using adjuncts to direct laryngoscopy • Using an alternative device or technique following failed intubation with direct laryngoscopy	Any 1	*The Cormack and Lehane grades 3 and 4 relate to difficult laryngoscopy, as opposed to a 'difficult airway'.*
b	• Inexperienced operator • Impending airway obstruction (at risk of 'cork-in-bottle') • Allergy to local anaesthetic agents • Infection/contamination of the upper airway: blood, friable tumour, open abscess • Grossly distorted anatomy • Fractured base of skull (contraindication to nasal route) • Penetrating eye injury • Uncooperative patient	Any 4	*AFOI may not be the best option if there is a potential to cause complete airway obstruction; the so-called cork-in-bottle situation, e.g. in glottic tumours where the aperture of the airway may be greatly reduced.* *AFOI in patients with an obstructed airway remains controversial – NAP 4 reported failure of this technique in 14 out of 23 head and neck cases.*

(cont.)

Q	Marking guidance	Mark	Comments
c	• Cricothyroid → tenses vocal cords • Thyroarytenoid and vocalis → slacken vocal cords • Lateral cricoarytenoid and transverse arytenoids → adduction of vocal cords • Posterior cricoarytenoid → abduction of vocal cords	4	*The extrinsic laryngeal muscles are responsible for movement of the larynx as a whole.* *The intrinsic laryngeal muscles (the transverse and oblique arytenoids and aryepiglottic muscles) adjust the aperture of the larynx.*
d	• Recurrent laryngeal supplies all laryngeal muscles with the exception of cricothyroid muscle	1	*The recurrent laryngeal nerve is a branch of the vagus nerve, with the right and left recurrent laryngeal nerves following differing paths. The recurrent laryngeal nerve provides sensation to the subglottis.*
	• External laryngeal nerve supplies the cricothyroid muscle	1	*The external and internal laryngeal nerves arise from the superior laryngeal nerve, which itself arises from the vagus nerve. The internal branch is the sensory supply to the glottis, supraglottis and inferior epiglottis.*
e	9 mg/kg	1	*Based on lean body mass, for adults >50 kg.* *The maximum dose in children is lower, up to 4.5 mg/kg.*
f	25% (accept 20%–30%)	1	
g	• Use of 21–23 G needle to pierce the cricothyroid membrane • Aspiration of air to confirm the tip of the needle is within the trachea	Any 4	*The resultant cough aids the spread of the local anaesthetic within the tracheobronchial tree.*

(cont.)

Q	Marking guidance	Mark	Comments
	• Injection (ideally whilst patient exhaling) of lignocaine • Trans-tracheal lignocaine dose calculated taking into account the lignocaine already administered to topicalise the supraglottic airway • Rapid removal of needle to ensure no trauma when the patient coughs		
h	• Airway equipment for re-intubation on standby • Extubation in theatre with trained assistant • Appropriate anaesthetic drugs drawn up in the required doses in case of need for resedation/intubation • Verbalised management strategy in case of failed extubation • Surgical team remain in operating theatre until successful extubation has been established • A period of observation in theatre, before transfer to recovery	Any 4	*The Difficult Airway Society guidelines recommend the following to optimise 'patient' factors:* • *Ensure cardiovascular stability* • *Ensure respiratory stability* • *Ensure metabolic/temperature stability* • *Ensure neuromuscular function has returned* *A 'cuff-leak' test is sometimes used to determine the relative safety of extubation – there is limited evidence for its value and it has not been shown to accurately predict post-extubation stridor. Given the topicalistion of her airway, Jennifer should be kept nil by mouth post-operatively until her risk of aspiration has returned to baseline.*

Suggested reading

S. Kritzinger, M Van Greunen. World Federation of Societies of Anaesthesiologists' Anaesthesia Tutorial of the Week 201. 2010. www.aagbi.org/sites/default/files/201-Awake-fibreoptic-intubation-the-basics.pdf. (Accessed 12 October 2018).

M. Morosan, A. Parbhoo. Anaesthesia and common oral and maxilla-facial emergencies. *Cont Edu Anaesth Crit Care Pain* 2012; **12**(5): 257–62.

Question 11   Mental Capacity and Deprivation of Liberties

Q	Marking guidance	Mark	Comments
a	• Alzheimer's disease • Vascular dementia (accept multi-infarct dementia) • Lewy body dementia	Any 2	
b	• Understand the decision to be made and the information given	1	
	• Retain the information long enough to make the decision	1	
	• Weigh up the information given	1	
	• Communicate their decision	1	
c	Assessment of best interests should include the following factors: • Social • Psychological • Medical • Should be the least burdensome option • Should be informed by the patient's attitudes and opinions	Any 4	*Family or close friends should be consulted to establish these factors for this patient.*
d	• Advanced directive/living will • Lasting Power of Attorney for Health and Welfare • Court-appointed deputy	Any 2	
e	Diagnosis: Post-operative delirium	1	
	Risk factors: • Previous delirium • Dementia • Age > 70 years • Alcohol abuse • Visual impairment • Hearing impairment • Hypertension • Vascular surgery • Depression • Severe illness/major surgery	Any 4	

(cont.)

Q	Marking guidance	Mark	Comments
f	That a person: • Is confined to a restricted place for a non-negligible period of time • Lacks capacity to consent to their care • Is subject to continuous and complete supervision and control • Is not free to leave	Any 2	*A DoLS application is not required in the majority of critical care situations, as stemmed from the 2017 P vs Cheshire West case.*
g	Independent Mental Capacity Advocate (IMCA)	1	*A medical decision can be made 'in best interests' if there is insufficient time to involve an IMCA.*

Suggested reading

T. Orr, R. Baruah. Consent in anaesthesia, critical care and pain medicine. *BJA Educ* 2018; **18**(5): 135–9.

S. Deiner, J. H. Silverstein. Postoperative delirium and cognitive dysfunction. *Br J Anaesth* 2009; **103**(Suppl.): i41–6.

Question 12 Free Flap Surgery

Q	Marking guidance	Mark	Comments
a	Hagen–Poiseuille equation: Blood flow $= \frac{\Delta P \pi r^4}{8 \eta l}$	1	One mark for correct equation, 1 mark for two correct factors, 2 marks for four correct factors.
	where ΔP is the pressure difference between the two ends of a tube r = radius of tube η = viscosity of fluid l = length of tube	2	
b	Viscosity is not constant, but varies with • Flow rates • Temperature • Haematocrit	3	*At low flow rates, viscosity increases – red blood cells aggregate into stacks (rouleaux formation).* *Hypothermia increases viscosity.* *A haematocrit of 0.3 is considered optimal.*
c	• Maintaining normothermia • Normovolaemia • Anaesthetic agents • Sympathetic blockade • Minimise surgical handling of flap NB Pharmacological vasodilatation is rarely used, due to steal phenomenon from a maximally dilated flap circulation.	Any 4	*Hypothermia causes both vasoconstriction and an increase in viscosity.* *Hypovolaemia causes vasoconstriction.* *Propofol and volatile anaesthetics all cause vasodilatation.* *Epidural or paravertebral blocks.* *Excessive surgical handling may precipitate vasospasm of the transplanted vessels.*

(cont.)

Q	Marking guidance	Mark	Comments
d	**Surgical:** • Arterial – vessel trauma, spasm, thrombus, technical problems with anastomosis • Venous – kinking of pedicle at anastomosis, spasm, thrombus, compression due to haematoma/dressings • Reperfusion injury due to prolonged ischaemic time **Non-surgical:** • Oedema due to excess fluid administration • Hypercoagulable state	Any 2 2	
e	• Evaluation of flap colour • Capillary refill time • Skin turgor • Skin temperature • Bleeding on pinprick • Transcutaneous Doppler signal over perforator artery	6	*Arterial ischaemia results in a cool, pale flap with slow capillary refill time, no bleeding on pinprick and loss of triphasic Doppler signal. In contrast, venous ischaemia results in a warm, congested, blue flap with short capillary refill time, rapid bleeding on pinprick and loss of venous Doppler signal.*

Suggested reading

N. Nimalan, O. A. Branford, G. Stocks. Anaesthesia for free flap breast reconstruction. *BJA Educ* 2016; **16**(5): 162–6.

J. Adams, P. Charlton. Anaesthesia for microvascular free tissue transfer. *BJA CEPD Rev* 2003; **3**(2): 33–7.

Paper 4 Answers

Question 1 Subarachnoid Haemorrhage

Q	Marking guidance	Mark	Comments
a	• Rupture of berry aneurysm • Rupture of arterio-venous malformation (AVM) • Traumatic subarachnoid haemorrhage (SAH)	1 1 1	*AVM rupture and traumatic subarachnoid account for 10% each, with aneurysm rupture accounting for 80% of subarachnoid haemorrhage.*
b	• Genetic • Associated conditions, e.g. polycystic kidneys • Smoking • Cocaine use • Amphetamine use • Ehlers–Danlos type IV	Any 4	*Familial risk is significant if a first-degree relative has SAH.*
c	i = Anterior cerebral artery ii = Anterior communicating artery iii = Middle cerebral artery iv = Posterior cerebral artery v = Basilar artery vi = Posterior communicating artery	3	No half marks, 1 mark for two correct answers.
d	• Anterior communicating artery • Middle cerebral artery • Posterior communicating artery	3	*Berry aneurysms occur at bifurcations of major arteries.*
e	• Hunt and Hess grading scale for subarachnoid haemorrhage (clinical) • WFNS Grading Scale for Aneurysmal Subarachnoid Haemorrhage (clinical) • Fisher grade (based on CT scan)	3	WFNS = World Federation of Neurological Surgeons *There are many more scoring systems, but these three are by far the most commonly used.*

Q	Marking guidance	Mark	Comments
f	Early: • Re-bleeding • Seizure • Hydrocephalus	Any 2	*Aneurysms are coiled or clipped within the first few days to prevent re-bleeding.*
	Late: • Delayed cerebral ischaemia/ vasospasm • Cognitive impairment • Neurocognitive symptoms such as fatigue, mood disturbance • Hypopituitarism	Any 2	*The highest risk period is 7–10 days following bleed. Nimodipine is taken for 21 days to reduce risk. Neuropsychiatric symptoms are common following SAH.*

Suggested reading

A. Luoma, U. Reddy. Acute management of aneurysmal subarachnoid haemorrhage. *Cont Edu Anaesth Crit Care Pain* 2013; **13**(2): 52–8.

Question 2   Congenital Heart Disease

Q	Marking guidance	Mark	Comments
a	• Sepsis • Hypoglycaemia • Metabolic/endocrine disorder • Trauma/non-accidental injury	Any 2	*The differential diagnosis of collapse in a neonate is broad. This is a critical time for the circulation: ductus arteriosus closure may unmask congenital heart disease.*
b	• Tachypnoea and sweating whilst feeding • Persistent tachycardia • Hepatomegaly • Oedema of face/forearm/back/legs • Radio-femoral delay • Cyanosis, especially on crying • Pathological murmur NB features of the history are not clinical signs	Any 4	*A history of feeding difficulty is common. Breathing and feeding cannot happen simultaneously, so cyanotic episodes are often precipitated by feeding.*
c	• Right ventricular outflow tract obstruction/pulmonary valve stenosis • Ventricular septal defect (VSD) • Right ventricular hypertrophy • Overriding aorta	1 1 1 1	
d	• DiGeorge syndrome • 22q11 chromosome deletion syndrome • Down's syndrome • Cleft lip/palate • Hypospadias	Any 2	
e	• Tachycardia • Hypotension • Defaecation • Crying	Any 2	

Q	Marking guidance	Mark	Comments
f	• Tet spell is usually precipitated by an acute decrease in systemic vascular resistance (SVR) • Or an acute increase in pulmonary vascular resistance (PVR) • → Increased right-to-left shunt across VSD • → Decreased P_aO_2/increased P_aCO_2, decreased pH • → Tachypnoea • → Increased negative intrathoracic pressure • → Increased venous return • → Increased right-to-left shunt across VSD • → Vicious cycle	Any 4	Maximum 4 marks
g	• Administer oxygen	Any 2	*The objective is to increase SVR, correct hypoxia and correct acidaemia. Oxygen administration decreases PVR.*
	• Console child in knee–chest position		*This is the equivalent of the older TOF child's squatting – increasing SVR.*
	• Opioids/ketamine/midazolam		*Relieves stress and hypercapnoea, but may decrease SVR.*
	• Correct any underlying cause, e.g. arrhythmia, hypothermia, hypoglycaemia		

Suggested reading

M. C. White, J. M. Peyton. Anaesthetic management of children with congenital heart disease for non-cardiac surgery. *Cont Edu Anaesth Crit Care Pain*, 2012; **12**(1): 17–22.

C. Apitz, G. D. Webb, A. N. Redington. Tetralogy of Fallot. *Lancet* 2009; **374**(9699): 1462–71.

Question 3 Diabetic Ketoacidosis

Q	Marking guidance	Mark	Comments
a	• Blood glucose > 11 mmol/L (accept > 13.9 mmol/L)	1	*As per the Joint British Societies Group.*
	• Ketonaemia > 3.0 mmol/L	1	*(The American Diabetes Association has slightly different guidance.)*
	• Bicarbonate < 15.0 mmol/L (accept < 18.0 mmol/L)	1	*A pH < 7.30 can be used in place of bicarbonate in the diagnostic criteria.*
b	Hyperglycaemia: • Lack of insulin-facilitated glucose uptake to muscles • Increase in antagonistic hormones (glucagon, cortisol, growth hormone) • Enhanced hepatic gluconeogenesis and glycogenolysis	Any 1	
	Ketonaemia: • Enhanced lipolysis increases free fatty acids • Fatty acids undergo β-oxidation into ketoacids	Any 1	
	Acidosis: • Ketoacids dissociate, releasing hydrogen ions • High anion gap metabolic acidosis	Any 1	
	Glycosuria: • Plasma glucose concentration exceeds capacity of proximal convoluted tubule to completely reabsorb glucose from filtrate	1	
c	• 10 mL of 10% calcium gluconate • 10 mL of 10% calcium chloride (accept 10–20 mL)	Any 1	*Immediate management also includes 50 mL of 50% dextrose together with 10 units of soluble insulin.*

(cont.)

Q	Marking guidance	Mark	Comments
d	• Peaked T waves • Prolonged PR segment • Loss of P-wave • Prolonged QRS complex • ST-segment elevation • Ectopic beats and escape rhythm • Widening of QRS complex • Sine wave • Ventricular fibrillation • Asystole • Axis deviation • Bundle branch block	Any 5	*A vast array of ECG changes may be seen in hyperkalaemia. They are normally classified as mild (5.5–6.5 mmol/L), moderate (6.5–7.5 mmol/L), and severe (>7.5 mmol/L), although classifications vary.* *Calcium reduces the excitability of cardiomyocytes, reducing the risk of fatal arrhythmias.*
e	• Hypokalaemia • Hypoglycaemia • Renal impairment • Cerebral oedema • Pulmonary oedema • Death	Any 4	*Insulin administration may cause hypokalaemia and hypoglycaemia. Fluid administration has been postulated to cause cerebral and pulmonary oedema.*
f	• 3-β-hydroxybutyrate • Acetoacetate • Acetone	3	*The predominant ketone in the body is 3-β-hydroxybutyrate, which is measured in point-of-care testing.*

Suggested reading

Joint British Societies Inpatient Care Group. The Management of Diabetic Ketoacidosis in Adults, 2nd edn, 2013. www.diabetes.org.uk/resources-s3/2017–09/Management-of-DKA-241013.pdf. (Accessed 6 September 2018).

Question 4 Pyloric Stenosis

Q	Marking guidance	Mark	Comments
a	• General condition: abnormally sleepy/lethargic • Anterior fontanelle: markedly sunken/depressed • Weak rapid pulse • Rapid respiratory rate • Urine output: <0.5 ml/kg/h • Skin turgor: decreased with tenting • Mucous membranes: very dry • Eyes: markedly sunken	Any 4	*Dehydration is classified in the context of fluid loss as a percentage of body weight.* *Mild = 5%* *Moderate = 10%* *Severe = 15%* *The classification can help guide fluid resuscitation.*
b	Hypokalaemic, hypochloraemic metabolic alkalosis (NB must state all three components for the mark)	1	*Whilst PCO_2 is raised, which may represent partial respiratory compensation, conclusions cannot easily be drawn due to this being a venous rather than an arterial blood sample.*
c	• More common in boys • Young maternal age • Maternal family history • Infants born in autumn and spring • Maternal smoking • Postnatal erythromycin • Association with bottle feeding	Any 4	*4:1 male:female ratio, especially common in first-born boys.*
d	• Visible peristalsis • Olive-like 2–3 cm palpable mass in right side of epigastrium	2	*Crossing abdomen from left to right.* *This clinical sign is less frequently found due to earlier diagnosis using ultrasound.*

(cont.)

Q	Marking guidance	Mark	Comments
e	• Antidiuretic hormone (ADH)	2	*By the hypothalamus/ posterior pituitary in response to increased plasma osmolarity.*
	• Renin Not acceptable: aldosterone, as it is secreted as an **indirect** response to increased renin secretion		*Secreted in response to decreased tubular filtrate flow rate or decreased perfusion of the macula densa.*
f	Aldosterone	1	*Acts at principle cells in the DCT and collecting ducts to absorb water and Na^+ in exchange for K^+ and H^+. In severe dehydration, the conservation of water takes precedence over normalising plasma pH.*
g	• Risk of aspiration on induction, but rapid sequence induction/ cricoid pressure difficult in this age group	Any 6	
	• Nasogastric or orogastric tube insertion and 'four quadrant' aspiration		*I.e. aspirating the tube with the infant supine, left lateral decubitus, prone and right lateral decubitus.*
	• Use a 3.5 mm cuffed or uncuffed endotracheal tube • Temperature control: increase the theatre ambient temperature to 26°C, use radiant heaters/forced air warmers • Analgesia provided using local anaesthetic techniques and paracetamol • Maintain normoglycaemia in the perioperative period: use of glucose-containing maintenance fluid		

(cont.)

Q	Marking guidance	Mark	Comments
	• Apnoea monitoring in a high-dependency environment		*Mandatory for infants < 44 weeks post-conceptual age, or for ex-premature infants < 60 weeks post post-conceptual age.*
	• Reduced IV paracetamol dose: 7.5 mg/kg every 6 hours for post-conceptual age 36–44 weeks		

Suggested reading

D. Fell, S. Chelliah. Infantile pyloric stenosis.
  BJA CEPD Reviews 2001; **1**(3): 85–8.

Question 5   Placenta Praevia

Q	Marking guidance	Mark	Comments
a	Grade 1: does not abut the internal cervical os/low-lying	1	*Placenta praevia has also been classified as minor or major.*
	Grade 2: reaches margin of internal cervical os/marginal	1	*Only 10% of those with a low-lying placenta at the 20-week scan will go on to have placenta praevia.*
	Grade 3: partially covers internal os/partial	1	
	Grade 4: completely covers internal cervical os/complete	1	
b	• Previous placenta praevia • Previous termination of pregnancy • Multiparity • Advanced maternal age (>40 years) • Smoking • Deficient endometrium – scarring, endometritis, manual removal of placenta, curettage, fibroid • Assisted conception • Previous caesarean section	Any 5	*In women who have previously had a caesarean section, 50% of those with a low-lying placenta at 20 weeks' gestation will go on to have placenta praevia.*
c	• Senior input – consultant anaesthetist • Additional monitoring – arterial line • Additional large bore intravenous access • Regional anaesthesia (must qualify association with reduced blood loss) • Consider general anaesthesia, or consent for rapid conversion • Cell salvage • Cross-match • Rapid infusor • Tranexamic acid • Consent for blood transfusion	Any 7	*Women with a placental edge < 2cm from the internal os are likely to be delivered by caesarean section. If uncomplicated, this is usually after 38 weeks' gestation.* *In women with a history of caesarean section and an anterior low-lying placenta, the risk of placenta accreta should be considered.*

(cont.)

Q	Marking guidance	Mark	Comments
d	Least common: placenta percreta	1	
	Intermediate: placenta increta	1	
	Most common: placenta accreta	1	
	Correct order of increasing incidence	1	

Suggested reading

F. Plaat, A. Shonfeld. Major obstetric haemorrhage. *Cont Edu Anaesth Crit Care Pain* 2015; **15**(4): 190–3.

Royal College of Obstetrics and Gynaecology. Placenta praevia, placenta praevia accreta and vasa praevia: diagnosis and management – Green-top Guideline No. 27. 2011. www.rcog.org.uk/en/guidelines-research-services/guidelines/gtg27a. (Accessed 22 October 2018).

Question 6 Post-herpetic Neuralgia

Q	Marking guidance	Mark	Comments
a	Varicella zoster virus (VZV) (accept human herpes virus type III)	1	*Following a primary infection with VZV (chickenpox), the virus lies dormant in spinal and cranial nerve ganglia.*
b	• Thoracic dermatome • Ophthalmic division of trigeminal nerve (ophthalmic division must be specified)	1 1	
c	• Diseases affecting the immune system, e.g. lymphoma, human immunodeficiency virus (HIV) • Pharmacological immunosuppression: e.g. following organ transplant, autoimmune disease • Treatment of malignancy: chemotherapy, radiotherapy	1 1 1	*Cell-mediated immunity normally prevents reactivation, but inhibition of the immune system may allow reactivation of VZV, causing the characteristic rash of shingles.*
d	• Age > 60 years • Female • More intense initial pain • More severe rash • Prodrome of dermatomal pain before development of rash • Fever (>38°C)	Any 4	

(cont.)

Q	Marking guidance	Mark	Comments
e	• Prodromal pain in a single dermatome before onset of rash	1	
	Pain: • Continuous or intermittent • Throbbing or burning • Allodynia – unable to wear clothing over the involved region	Any 2	
	Other neurological: • Sensory loss • Motor weakness • Autonomic disturbance – abnormal skin temperature/colour, abnormal sweating	Any 3	
	Psychological symptoms: • Isolation • Depression/anxiety • Chronic fatigue • Sleep disturbance	Any 2	
	Systemic symptoms: • Weight loss	1	
f	• VZV vaccine booster • Antiviral drugs: acyclovir, valaciclovir, famciclovir	Any 1	*Antiviral drugs shorten the period of viral replication, and halve the incidence of PHN at 6 months.*
g	• Simple analgesics: paracetamol ± codeine • Gabapentinoids: gabapentin, pregabalin • Tricyclic antidepressants • Topical agents: lignocaine and capsacin • Weak opioids: tramadol	Any 3	

Suggested reading

R. Gupta, P. F. Smith. Post-herpetic neuralgia. *Cont Edu Anaesth Crit Care Pain* 2012; **12**(4): 181–5.

National Institute for Care and Health Excellence Clinical Knowledge Summary: Post-herpetic neuralgia. 2017. http://cks.nice.org.uk/post-herpetic-neuralgia. (Accessed 16 August 2018).

Question 7 Parathyroidectomy

Q	Marking guidance	Mark	Comments
a	• Bone pain • Muscle weakness, reduced reflexes • Fatigue Gastrointestinal: • Constipation • Anorexia • Nausea and vomiting Renal: • Polyuria resulting in dehydration • Renal stones Neuropsychiatric: • Depression/anxiety • Cognitive dysfunction: confusion, psychosis • Insomnia	Any 6	*The classical description of 'stones, bones, abdominal groans and psychic moans' is rarely seen, with the majority of patients having few symptoms on diagnosis.* *The mechanism of polyuria is nephrogenic diabetes insipidus secondary to nephrocalcinosis.* *Depression is common, up to 40% of patients are affected.*
b	• Two pairs of parathyroid glands • Embedded in the superior and inferior poles of the thyroid gland bilaterally	1 1	*There is considerable variability in the number of glands and their location. The parathyroid glands may even descend into the thorax with the thymus.*
c	Technetium-99 m-sestamibi scintigraphy	1	*Accept 'nuclear medicine scan'*
d	Kidney: • Increased Ca^{2+} resorption in the loop of Henle, distal convoluted tubule and collecting duct • Increased phosphate (PO_4^{3-}) excretion in the proximal convoluted tubule	Max 2	

(cont.)

Q	Marking guidance	Mark	Comments
	• Increased production of 1,25-dihydroxycholecalciferol (vitamin D_3)		*PTH increases the activity of 1-α-hydroxylase enzyme, which converts 25-hydroxycholecalciferol to vitamin D_3.*
	Bone:		
	• Increased bone resorption to release Ca^{2+}	1	
	• Inhibits osteoblast activity, stimulates osteoclasts activity	1	
	Intestine:		
	• Ca^{2+} is reabsorbed indirectly	1	*The PTH-induced increase in vitamin D is responsible for this effect.*
e	• Lower doses of anaesthetic agents may be needed if somnolent	Any 2	*The risk of intra-operative cardiac arrhythmias is much greater for patients with $Ca^{2+} > 3.0$ mmol/L.*
	• Hypercalcaemia may augment neuromuscular blockade: reduce doses of muscle relaxants and use neuromuscular monitoring		
	• Increased incidence of cardiac arrhythmias		
f	• Peri-oral/digital parasthesias	Any 4	
	• Positive Trousseau's sign		*Trousseau's sign is inducing carpal spasm by inflating a blood pressure cuff.*
	• Positive Chvostek's sign		
	• Carpopedal spasm		
	• Laryngospasm		*Chvostek's sign is facial spasm induced by tapping the inferior zygoma.*
	• ECG changes: prolonged QT interval and torsades de pointes		*Mnemonic for severe hypocalcaemia: CATS go numb = convulsions, arrythmias, tetany, laryngospasm, go numb = paraesthesias.*
	• Negative chronotropy/inotropy		

(cont.)

Q	Marking guidance	Mark	Comments
g	• Multiple endocrine neoplasia (MEN) type 1 and 2A • Familial isolated hyperparathyroidism	Any 1	*The multiple endocrine neoplasias are syndromes characterised by tumours of several endocrine glands. MEN 1 is characterised by the '3Ps' – pituitary, parathyroid and pancreatic – MEN 2A by '2Ps and 1 M': phaeochromocytoma, parathyroid, medullary thyroid.*

Suggested reading

P. Sasidharan, I. G. Johnston. Parathyroid physiology and anaesthesia. World Federation of Societies of Anaesthesiologists' Anaesthesia Tutorial of the Week 142. 2009. www.aagbi.org/sites/default/files/142-anaesthesia-the-parathyroid-gland.pdf. (Accessed 17 August 2018).

S. Malhotra, V. Sodhi. Anaesthesia for thyroid and parathyroid surgery. *Cont Edu Anaesth Crit Care Pain* 2007; **7**(2): 55–8.

M. Parikh, S. T. Webb. Cations: potassium, calcium, and magnesium. *Cont Edu Anaesth Crit Care Pain* 2012; **12**(4): 195–8.

Question 8   Oesophageal Rupture

Q	Marking guidance	Mark	Comments
a	• Chest/neck surgical emphysema • Resonant percussion • Dull percussion • Reduced air entry on auscultation • Hamman crunch	Any 4	*Due to pneumothorax.* *Due to atelectasis or consolidation.* *Due to atelectasis or consolidation.* *Cracking sound of pneumomediastinum on auscultation.*
b	• Peri-oesophageal air • Pneumomediastinum • Pneumopericardium • Cervical surgical emphysema • Pneumothorax • Pleural effusion (usually left sided) • Lung abscess • Pneumoperitoneum	Any 4	*Which tissues are contaminated by air/gastric contents depends on the location of the oesophageal perforation. Boerhaave syndrome most commonly affects the mid-thoracic oesophagus, whilst trauma secondary to oesophagoscopy most commonly results in perforation at the cricopharyngeus, and just proximal to the lower oesophageal sphincter.*
c	• Sepsis is likely with potential for haemodynamic instability – consider use of cardiostable induction agent, e.g. ketamine	1	
	• Rapid sequence induction is indicated, but suxamethonium increases intragastic pressure – use rocuronium	1	*The use of cricoid pressure (which may increase the risk of exacerbating mediastinal contamination through coughing/ straining) must be balanced against the risk of soiling lungs.*

(cont.)

Q	Marking guidance	Mark	Comments
d	• Double-lumen endotracheal tube (DLETT)	1	*Left sided DLETT is usually preferred, as right-sided DLETT risks occlusion of the right upper lobe bronchus.*
	• Single lumen endotracheal tube with bronchial blocker	1	*An endotracheal tube of at least 7.5 mm is required.*
e	• Low tidal volume: 6–8 mL/kg during two lung ventilation, 5–6 mL/kg whilst on one-lung ventilation	Any 2	
	• Permissive hypercapnoea		
	• Avoid fluid overload		*Fluid guided by pulse contour analysis cardiac output monitor – clearly this is not the time to use an oesophageal Doppler!*
f	• Displacement of double-lumen endotracheal tube	Any 6	*A fibre-optic scope should be immediately available, and the DLETT position checked following any patient repositioning.*
	• $\dot{V}/\dot{Q}$ mismatch and shunt, leading to hypoxaemia		
	• Radial nerve palsy in superior arm		*The radial nerve is particularly at risk if the arm is abducted > 90°; an axillary roll is used to prevent mid-humeral radial nerve compression.*
	• Common perineal nerve palsy in the inferior leg		*Due to compression between the fibular head and the operating table.*
	• Saphenous nerve palsy of either leg		*A pillow is usually placed between the knees to prevent this complication.*
	• Brachial plexus injury		*The neck must be in a neutral position to prevent brachial plexus stretch.*

(cont.)

Q	Marking guidance	Mark	Comments
	• Ear injury		*Ensure that the ear has not folded during positioning.*
	• Optic neuropathy		*The lower globe is at risk from external compression from the pillow in the lateral position.*
	• Pressure injury to bony prominences, e.g. iliac crest		

Suggested reading

W. D. King, M. C. Dickinson. Oesophageal injury. *BJA Educ* 2015; **15**(5): 265–70.

Question 9 Obesity and Laparoscopy

Q	Marking guidance	Mark	Comments
a	• Obesity class III	1	*According to the WHO classification of obesity 2014. This BMI would previously have been classified as morbidly obese.*
b	• Craniofacial abnormalities (such as Pierre–Robin and Down's syndromes) • Tonsillar and adenoidal hypertrophy • Male gender • Age 40–70 years • Enlarged neck circumference • Neuromuscular disease	Any 4	*= the major cause of OSA in children.* *Male gender: possibly as a result of a relatively increased amount of fat deposition around the pharynx.* *>37 cm women,* *>43 cm men.*
c	• Neuropsychiatric: depression, anxiety • Endocrinological: diabetes mellitus, dyslipidaemia, infertility, hypothyroidism • Cardiovascular: hypertension, myocardial infarction, stroke, atrial fibrillation, pulmonary hypertension (accept up to two cardiovascular conditions, and one from each of the other categories)	1 1 Max 2	*OSA patients experience many neuropsychiatric symptoms such as daytime somnolence, impaired concentration, irritability. These are not considered 'health conditions'.*

(cont.)

Q	Marking guidance	Mark	Comments
d	• Weight loss • Reduce/stop alcohol intake • Smoking cessation • Nasal continuous positive airway pressure (nCPAP) • Sleep modification (i.e. sleeping in lateral position or 30° head up instead of supine)	Any 4	*Overnight nCPAP set at between +5 and +20 cmH$_2$O probably works by acting as a pneumatic splint to maintain upper airway patency. It has the effect of reducing daytime sleepiness, improving mood and cognitive function, and improving blood pressure control.*
e	• Increased systemic vascular resistance	Any 4	*This is thought to be due to mechanical compression of the aorta, release of vasoactive substances – vasopressin, catecholamines, and activation of the renin-angiotensin-aldosterone system.*
	• Decreased preload due to compression of the inferior vena cava		
	• Diaphragmatic splinting/reduced functional residual capacity		*Results in atelectasis and $\dot{V}/\dot{Q}$ mismatch*
	• Raised intrathoracic pressure/reduced pulmonary compliance		
	• Decreased liver/renal/splanchnic arterial and venous blood flow		*Glomerular filtration rate decreases by ~25%; gut mucosal blood flow decreases by ~40%.*
	• Decreased cerebral venous drainage, which leads to raised intracranial pressure		*This is of particular relevance for prolonged surgical procedures performed in a steep Trendelenburg position, which may result in cerebral oedema.*

(cont.)

Q	Marking guidance	Mark	Comments
	• Activation of the sympathetic nervous system ± parasympathetic nervous system		
f	• Manual handling of the patient	Any 4	*Greater number of members of staff required for lateral transfer, plus special equipment (e.g. hover mattress).*
	• Width of operating table		*Side extensions are often required for bariatric patients.*
	• Patient movement on operating table once positioned in reverse Trendelenburg		*Bariatric patients are often positioned prior to induction of anaesthesia in a seated position with a support under bent knees to limit movement.*
	• Reduced venous return in reverse Trendelenburg position		*In combination with pneumoperitoneum may result in hypotension.*
	• Peripheral nerve injury		*This is a complication of surgical positioning in any patient, but particularly in the left arm following left lateral tilt.*

Suggested reading

P. Hayden, S. Cowman. Anaesthesia for laparoscopic surgery. *Cont Edu Anaesth Crit Care Pain* 2011; **11**(5): 177–80.

G. Martinez, P. Faber. Obstructive sleep apnoea. *Cont Edu Anaesth Crit Care Pain* 2011; **11**(1): 5–8.

Question 10 Bimaxillary Osteotomy

Q	Marking guidance	Mark	Comments
a	• Shared airway	Any 6	
	• Nasal intubation required		*The mouth must be free to enable the occlusion of the teeth to be checked intra-operatively.*
	• Nasal intubation risks epistaxis		*Due to direct trauma to Kisselbach's plexus of Little's area.*
	• Intra-operative damage to nasal endotracheal tube		*The site of surgery is in close proximity to the nasal tube.*
	• Bimaxillary surgery may be performed in patients with comorbidities associated with difficult laryngoscopy		*E.g. previous cleft palate repair, obstructive sleep apnoea.*
	• Possibility of patient being woken with rigid inter-maxillary fixation (IMF)		*IMF is 'wiring' the teeth together – more commonly, elastic bands are applied after the patient has left PACU.*
	• Intra-operative throat pack commonly used		
	• Intra-operative head movement may result in extubation or endobronchial intubation		
	• Post-operative bleeding/ haematoma		*Post-operative bleeding may rapidly result in airway obstruction, particularly in patients with rigid IMF.*
b	• Retromolar reinforced oral endotracheal tube	3	*An oral flexible endotracheal tube is pushed behind the molar teeth, so that the teeth can still be occluded.*
	• Submental intubation		*The end of a conventional endotracheal tube (minus its connector) is passed through the floor of the mouth.*
	• Tracheostomy		

Q	Marking guidance	Mark	Comments
c	• Position the patient head up • Induced hypotension • Surgical infiltration with adrenaline-containing local anaesthetic • Tranexamic acid	4	*The bony mid-face receives an extensive blood supply, and the posterior maxilla is close to the pterygoid venous plexus.*
d	• Reduced incidence of post-operative nausea and vomiting (PONV) • Used to induce intra-operative hypotension, improving operative field • Smooth extubation without coughing or straining	3	*PONV is common in bimaxillary osteotomy surgery, and may be dangerous if jaws are wired post-operatively.* *Coughing and straining may promote bleeding.*
e	• Label or mark the patient's head with an adherent sticker • Label the endotracheal tube or laryngeal mask airway • Attach the pack to the artificial airway • Leave part of the pack protruding • Include in the swab count • Not using a throat pack	Any 4	*Retained throat pack is a 'never event'. The National Patient Safety Agency issued a Safer Practice Notice with these recommendations in 2009.*

Suggested reading

J. I. Beck, K. D. Johnston. Anaesthesia for cosmetic and functional maxillofacial surgery. *Cont Edu Anaesth Crit Care Pain* 2014; **14**(1): 38–42.

Question 11 Magnetic Resonance Imaging

Q	Marking guidance	Mark	Comments
a	• Topical Eutectic Mixture of Local Anaesthetics (EMLA)/Ametop	4	*If accepted by the patient!*
	• Midazolam		*Oral/buccal (10–20 mg) has an unpleasant taste that can be masked with squash/juice; intranasal (0.2 mg/kg) stings.*
	• Temazepam		*Dose 10–30 mg, tablets may not be acceptable to the patient.*
	• Ketamine		*Side effects: increased salivation, dissociative state. Routes of administration are oral 5–10 mg/kg, intranasal 3–5 mg/kg, intramuscular 4 mg/kg.*
	• Clonidine		*Oral dose 4 µg/kg.*
b	• Hydrogen atoms are abundant within the body within water molecules	Any 4	
	• Hydrogen atoms possess a property called 'spin'		
	• When surrounded by a strong magnet, spin aligns with the magnetic field		
	• Spin can be turned out of alignment with the magnetic field by applying pulses of electromagnetic radiation		
	• The energy emitted is detected by three receiving coils, and translated into a series of grey pixels on a screen		*The three coils are positioned to generate a three-dimensional image.*

(cont.)

Q	Marking guidance	Mark	Comments
c	Superconductivity: • A phenomenon where electrical resistance in a coil of wire decreases to zero below a critical temperature	1	
	• Passing of an electric current through a coil of wire results in a strong magnetic field (electromagnet)	1	*A typical MR scanner uses a magnetic field strength of 1.5 Tesla.*
	Achieved by: • Cooled to 4.2 K by surrounding the coils in liquid helium	1	*This is usually surrounded by a jacket of liquid nitrogen, which has a boiling point of 77 K, to keep the expensive liquid helium from boiling away.*
d	• Cardiac pacemaker/loop recorder • Aneurysm clip • Cochlear implant • Shrapnel/penetrating eye injury involving metal • Cardiac defibrillator • Any type of nerve/neuro stimulator • Joint replacement • Hydrocephalus shunt	Any 4	
e	The pilot balloon	1	*The pilot balloon contains a ferromagnetic spring which is normally secured by tape, away from the area to be scanned.*

(cont.)

Q	Marking guidance	Mark	Comments
f	• Time-varying magnetic gradient fields	1	*Small dynamic magnetic fields can induce a current sufficient to stimulate peripheral nerve and muscle cells, causing discomfort.*
	• Acoustic noise	1	*Switching of gradient fields creates loud acoustic noise, above the safe level of 85 dB – patients and staff need ear protection.*
	• Radiofrequency heating	1	*Power dissipation within the patient, causing an increase in body temperature. There is a risk of severe, rapid burns from any conductive material left on the patient's skin: ECG leads, metal in clothing etc.*
	• Helium escape	1	*In the event of a spontaneous or emergency field shutdown (a 'quench'), the liquid helium (and nitrogen) expands to a gas and must be vented very rapidly, with the potential for a hypoxic environment within the MRI scan room.*

Suggested reading

U. Reddy, M. J. White, S. R. Wilson. Anaesthesia for magnetic resonance imaging. *Cont Edu Anaesth Crit Care Pain* 2012; **12**(3): 140–4.

Question 12 Airway Burns

Q	Marking guidance	Mark	Comments
a	• Singed hairs of eyebrows/ eyelashes/nasal hair • Swelling of the face, lips, tongue or uvula • Soot in nose/mouth/sputum • Inspiratory stridor • Change in voice/hoarseness • Dyspnoea • Coughing • Wheezing • Copious secretions	Any 5	*Inhalational injury is important to exclude because airway swelling may rapidly turn an easy intubation into an impossible intubation.*
b	First-degree burn: red, painful, dry, no blisters Second-degree burn: red, blistered, painful, oedematous Third-degree burn: white, painless, no bleeding on pricking with a needle	3	*Only epidermis involved.* *Epidermis and dermis involved.* *Full thickness burn causing destruction of all skin layers plus underlying tissues.*
c	• Wallace 'Rule of nines' (accept: Lund-Browder chart) • Chest/abdomen represents 18% BSA; one arm represents 9% BSA	1	*The adult head represents 9% BSA, whereas a child has a proportionally bigger head (representing 18% BSA) and smaller legs (representing 13.5% BSA each).*
d	Parkland formula: • Fluid requirement 4 mL × weight kg × % burn • Half of the fluid given within the first 8 hours, the other half over the next 16 hours. Prescription: 4 mL × 100 kg × 30% = 12,000 mL ⇒ Prescription: 6000 mL Hartmann's over 7 hours, then 6000 mL Hartmann's over 16 hours	1 1 2	*The Parkland formula is the most widely used in the UK. It does not incorporate maintenance fluid which should be considered in addition to the resuscitation fluid.*

(cont.)

Q	Marking guidance	Mark	Comments
e	• Age: < 5 years or > 60 years old • Site of burn: hands, feet, perineum, any flexure (e.g. neck, axilla), circumferential burn of limb, torso or neck. • Inhalational injury • Mechanism of burn: chemical, steam, ionising radiation • > 10% BSA burn (adult) or > 5% BSA burn (child) • Significant comorbidities • Significant associated injuries, e.g. head injury, crush injury	Any 3	*These are the British Burns Association referral criteria.*
f	• Rapid sequence induction • Uncut endotracheal tube • Tape the endotracheal tube in place rather than use a tie • Minimum of size 8.0 mm endotracheal tube to facilitate bronchoscopy • Insert a nasogastric tube at the same time	Any 3	*If inhalational injury is suspected, early intubation is crucial. The specialist burns centre will be happy to receive an intubated patient who they can extubate the following day if there are concerns about the airway.* *Suxamethonium is not contraindicated until 48 hours after the burn.*

Suggested reading

S. Bishop, S. Maguire. Anaesthesia and intensive care for major burns. *Cont Edu Anaesth Crit Care Pain* 2012; **12**(3): 118–22.

Paper 5 Answers

Question 1 Pituitary Disease

Q	Marking guidance	Mark	Comments
a	Bitemporal hemianopia	1	*Due to optic nerve compression at the optic chiasm.*
b	Diagnosis: Acromegaly/growth hormone-secreting pituitary macroadenoma	1	*In acromegaly, IGF-1 is chronically raised despite GH being elevated (IGF-1 should suppress GH secretion). Giving the patient a 75g glucose load should also suppress GH secretion.*
	Clinical features: • Coarsening of facial features (frontal bossing, enlarged nose/jaw/lips/ears, prognathism, increased interdental spacing, macroglossia) • Soft tissue changes (increased skin thickness, sweating, enlargement of hands and feet) • Carpal tunnel syndrome • Obstructive sleep apnoea • Sexual dysfunction (reduced libido, infertility, erectile dysfunction); oligomenorrhoea, galactorrhoea • Headache • Hypertension • Type II diabetes mellitus • Arthropathy • Cardiomegaly/cardiomyopathy • Vocal cord hypertrophy/deepening of voice	Any 5	Maximum 2 marks for facial features. *Often bilateral.* *Due to macroglossia and pharyngeal soft tissue growth.* *Usually due to prolactin co-secretion by the adenoma, or by prolactin secretion as the pituitary stalk is compressed by the adenoma.*

235

(cont.)

Q	Marking guidance	Mark	Comments
c	• ACTH triggered by hypothalamic CRH release • TSH triggered by hypothalamic TRH release • FSH triggered by hypothalamic GnRH release • LH triggered by hypothalamic GnRH release • GH triggered by hypothalamic GHRH release • PRL triggered by decrease in hypothalamic dopamine release	6	*Not acceptable: melanocyte stimulating hormone (MSH), as MSH is released from the intermediate lobe of the pituitary, located between the anterior and posterior lobes.* *The hormones released by the posterior pituitary are oxytocin and ADH.*
d	• Controlled hypercapnoea	1	*Increases cerebral blood flow and thus intracranial pressure, pushing the pituitary gland into the sella turcica.*
	• Injection of saline into a lumbar drain	1	*Increases lumbar CSF pressure, and thus intracranial pressure, again pushing the pituitary gland down into the sella turcica.*
e	<u>Endocrine complications:</u> • Diabetes insipidus	Any 2	*Usually resolves spontaneously, but if it persists patients will require long-term desmopressin.*
	• Adrenocortical deficiency		*Patients are routinely given a post-operative reducing regime of corticosteroids, adjusted according to post-operative hormonal function.*
	• Panhypopituitarism		*May occur following extensive pituitary resection; thyroid and sex hormone replacement will also be required.*

Q	Marking guidance	Mark	Comments
	Neurosurgical complications:	Any 2	
	• Cerebrospinal fluid leak/ rhinorrhoea		*This can be distinguished from mucous rhinorrhoea by testing nasal discharge with a dipstick for glucose.*
	• Vascular injury (internal carotid artery within the cavernous sinus)		*The cavernous sinus surrounds the pituitary gland.*
	• Optic nerve injury		
	• Nasal septum perforation		
	• Anosmia due to cribriform plate injury		
	• Post-operative sinusitis		
f	Colonoscopy	1	*High risk of colorectal carcinoma.*

Suggested reading

R. Menon. Anaesthesia and pituitary disease. *Cont Edu Anaesth Crit Care Pain* 2011; **11**(4): 133–7.

Question 2 Valvular Heart Disease

Q	Marking guidance	Mark	Comments
a	• Bicuspid aortic valve • Rheumatic heart disease • Paget's disease • Fabry's disease • Systemic lupus erythematosus	Any 2	
b	Severity: Mild: 1.2–1.8 cm^2 (accept 1.5–2.0 cm^2) Moderate: 0.8–1.2 cm^2 (accept 1.0–1.5 cm^2) Severe: 0.6–0.8 cm^2 (accept 0.6–1.0 cm^2) Critical: <0.6 cm^2	4	*The pressure gradient can also be used to describe severity of aortic stenosis, but severity is underestimated once the left ventricle starts to fail.* *Mild: 12–25 mmHg* *Moderate: 25–40 mmHg* *Severe: 40–50 mmHg* *Critical: >50 mmHg*
c	Principle → reasoning: • Maintain sinus rhythm → dependent on atrial contraction for ventricular filling • Avoid tachycardia/maintain heart rate < 90 beats/min → tachycardia reduces diastolic time and myocardial perfusion • Avoid bradycardia/maintain heart rate > 60 beats/min → heart rate dependent due to fixed stroke volume • Maintain diastolic blood pressure (DBP) → ensure adequate coronary perfusion pressure (CPP)	Any 8	One mark for each correct principle, up to 4 marks; 1 mark for each reasoning, up to 4 marks. *CPP = DBP − left ventricular end-diastolic pressure (LVEDP)*

Q	Marking guidance	Mark	Comments
	• Avoid reduction in systemic vascular resistance (SVR) → maintain blood pressure due to fixed cardiac output (CO)		*Patients with severe aortic stenosis have a fixed cardiac output. They cannot compensate for reductions in SVR – this will result in severe hypotension, impaired myocardial perfusion and subsequently reduced contractility.*
	• Avoid increases in SVR → increases myocardial workload/ O_2 requirement		
	• Maintain contractility/maintain cardiac output → relatively fixed stroke volume		*Remember:* *CO = HR × SV* *BP = CO × SVR*
d	• Heart block • Left axis deviation • ST depression/T-wave inversion in lateral leads (must specify leads) • P-wave enlargement	Any 2	*The aortic valve is very close to the atrioventricular node: calcification may result in heart block.*
e	Major: • Positive blood cultures • Positive echocardiogram finding defined as – Oscillating intracardiac mass – Intracardiac abscess – Partial dehiscence of prosthetic valve	Any 2	*'Positive echocardiogram' is not enough for a mark – there must be a defined finding as described.* *Infective endocarditis is an infrequent and dynamic disease.*
	Minor: • Predisposition (e.g. heart condition, IV drug use) • Fever • Vascular/immunological phenomena, such as: – Arterial emboli – Septic infarcts – Mycotic aneurysm	Any 2	*Despite modern medical and surgical therapy, it is still associated with high rates of complications and increased mortality. Early surgery is becoming more common, and a multidisciplinary team approach is vital.*

(cont.)

Q	Marking guidance	Mark	Comments
	– Intracranial haemorrhage – Conjunctival haemorrhages – Janeway lesions • Other microbiological evidence, such as PCR/serological tests		*Transoesophageal echocardiography should be used in all patients.*

Suggested reading

G. Martinez, K. Valchanov. Infective endocarditis. *Cont Edu Anaesth Crit Care Pain* 2012; **12**(3): 134–9.

J. Brown, N. J. Morgan-Hughes. Aortic stenosis and non-cardiac surgery. *Cont Edu Anaesth Crit Care Pain* 2005; **5**(1): 1–4.

Question 3   Critical Care Airway

Q	Marking guidance	Mark	Comments
a	20%–30%	1	*25% in NAP4*
b	• Aspiration risk: critical care patients are often not adequately fasted • Difficult airway: airway assessment is often challenging • Inadequate preoxygenation: the patient may already have significant hypoxaemia • Agitation/confusion may impair preoxygenation • Respiratory pathology, e.g. shunt/pulmonary infection causing $\dot{V}/\dot{Q}$ mismatch • Cardiovascular impairment: contributing to $\dot{V}/\dot{Q}$ mismatch • Difficult patient positioning	Any 6	*There are numerous reasons why airway interventions in critical care are more likely to be difficult. These can be categorised as* *1. Environmental/location factors, e.g. critical care is isolated from certain pieces of anaesthetic equipment.* *2. Patient factors, as discussed.* *3. Staff factors. Experience of assisting with smaller number of intubations means that critical care nursing staff tend to be relatively deskilled compared to anaesthetic assistants.*
c	Factors relating to the patient: <u>M</u>allampati class III or IV (score = 5) Obstructive sleep <u>A</u>pnoea syndrome (score = 2) Reduced mobility of <u>C</u>ervical spine (score = 1) Limited mouth <u>O</u>pening < 3 cm (score = 1) Factors relating to pathology: <u>C</u>oma (score = 1) Severe <u>H</u>ypoxaemia (SpO_2 < 80%) (score = 1) Factors relating to operator: Non-<u>A</u>naesthetist (score = 1)	Any 4	*The MACOCHA score comprises seven components in three domains, with a maximum score of 12. It is the only airway assessment score which has been validated in critically ill patients.*
	A MACOCHA score > 3 predicts difficult intubation in the critically ill	1	

(cont.)

Q	Marking guidance	Mark	Comments
d	• Long-term mechanical ventilation	Any 4	
	• Failed extubation/failure of weaning from the ventilator		*Prolonged weaning is often defined as weaning lasting longer than 7 days after the first spontaneous breathing trial.*
	• Upper airway obstruction • Difficult airway		*Cricothyroidotomy is preferred as an airway rescue technique as it is technically easier to perform and is associated with less bleeding.*
	• Need for airway access for tracheal toilet • Airway protection		
e	• Coagulopathy • Significant gas exchange deficiency (positive end-expiratory pressure ≥ 10 cmH$_2$O, fraction of inspired oxygen ≥ 0.6) • Infection at insertion site • Difficult anatomy (accept maximum of two from: short neck, cervical spine injury, limited neck movement, aberrant vessels, thyroid pathology)	4	

Suggested reading

A. Higgs, B. A. McGrath, C. Goddard, et al. Guidelines for the management of tracheal intubation in critically ill adults. *Br J Anaesth* 2018; **120**(2): 323–52.

Question 4 Cerebral Palsy

Q	Marking guidance	Mark	Comments
a	**Antenatal:** • Prematurity (<32 weeks gestation) • Multiple births • Low birth weight (<2.5 kg) • Intrauterine 'TORCH' infections: toxoplasmosis, varicella, rubella, cytomegalovirus, herpes (accept maternal infection) • Foetal alcohol syndrome • Congenital metabolic syndrome • Maternal hyperthyroidism **Postnatal:** • Neonatal jaundice/kernicterus • Birth complications: placental abruption, uterine rupture, pre-eclampsia, hypoxic injury • Events in the first 2 years of life: trauma, cerebral infection, cerebral haemorrhage/infarction, seizures	Any 2 Any 2	*Antenatal causes account for ~80% of cases of cerebral palsy.*
b	• Learning difficulties → pre-operative anxiety • Communication difficulties: expressive language disorders, motor problems affecting speech/visual/auditory impairment → difficult to communicate anxiety and pain • Epilepsy → antiepileptic drugs may cause enzyme induction/inhibition, reduce MAC by 30%, cause sedation/slower recovery from anaesthesia • Abnormal pain perception → post-operative pain may be difficult to manage • Spasticity → difficulty positioning	Any 3	One mark for each correct clinical feature; 1 mark for each corresponding anaesthetic implication. *Patients often take multiple antiepileptic drugs with long half-lives and a tendency to accumulate.*

(cont.)

Q	Marking guidance	Mark	Comments
c	• Gastro-oesophageal reflux → risk of aspiration pneumonia on induction of anaesthesia • Pseudo-bulbar palsy, leading to drooling and poor nutrition → dehydration, anaemia, electrolyte disturbance • Oesophageal dysmotility → aspiration pneumonia, poorly compliant chest	Any 2	*Overnight supplementation of nutrition via a nasogastric tube or PEG is common in this patient group. Surgical fundoplication may be required to control gastro-oesophageal reflux.*
d	• Repeated aspiration pneumonia → chronic lung disease/lung scarring • Prematurity → chronic lung disease secondary to infant respiratory distress syndrome • Scoliosis → restrictive lung deficit, pulmonary hypertension • Respiratory muscle hypotonia → poor cough, recurrent infection	Any 2	*Muscle spasms promote the development of scoliosis, which may ultimately lead to pulmonary hypertension and respiratory failure.*
e	Mechanism: GABA$_B$ receptor antagonist, inhibits release of aspartate and glutamate Site of action: Dorsal horn of spinal cord (Rex laminae II and III)	1 1	*Baclofen can be given orally or intrathecally through a subcutaneously implanted infusion device.*

Suggested reading

D. P. Prosser, N. Sharma. Cerebral palsy and anaesthesia. *Cont Edu Anaesth Crit Care Pain* 2010; **10**(3): 72–6.

Question 5 Post-dural Puncture Headache

Q	Marking guidance	Mark	Comments
a	• Frontal-occipital headache • Worse in the upright position • Positive Gutsche sign • Nuchal rigidity • Photophobia • Tinnitus • Visual disturbance • Cranial nerve palsies	Any 6	*The International Headache Society defines PDPH as one attributed to low cerebrospinal (CSF) pressure, developing within 5 days of neuraxial blockade and remitting spontaneously within 2 weeks or following an epidural blood patch. Gutsche sign is when right upper quadrant abdominal pressure results in temporary improvement of the headache.*
b	• Non-specific/tension headache • Migraine • Pre-eclampsia • Cortical vein thrombosis • Subarachnoid/subdural haemorrhage • Posterior reversible leukoencephalopathy syndrome • Space occupying lesion • Infection – encephalitis, meningitis, sinusitis	Any 6	*The mechanism of headache in PDPH is explained by the loss of CSF. This results in compensatory vasodilatation of cerebral vessels and leads to traction on the pain sensitive intracranial vasculature. Clinical features of serious pathology should always be sought.*
c	• Needle size: smaller gauge • Needle type: pencil point over Quincke • Re-insertion of stylet prior to removal of spinal needle • Experienced operator • Other techniques to optimise single pass success, such as optimal positioning, use of ultrasound	Any 4	*The incidence of PDPH following spinal anaesthesia has fallen due to the widespread adoption of smaller-gauge, pencil-point spinal needles.*

(cont.)

Q	Marking guidance	Mark	Comments
d	• Cerebral venous sinus thrombosis • Cranial nerve palsies • Subdural haematoma • Brainstem compression • Death • Persistent CSF leak/chronic headache/intracranial hypotension	Any 4	*A recent MBRRACE report highlighted two deaths in women with PDPH, although both cases were related to inadvertent dural puncture during epidural insertion.* *All patients with PDPH should be followed up, regardless of management.*

Suggested reading

A. Sabharwal, G. M. Stocks. Postpartum headache: diagnosis and management. *Cont Edu Anaesth Crit Care Pain* 2011; **11**(5): 181–5.

D. K. Turnbull, D. B. Shepherd. Post-dural puncture headache: pathogenesis, prevention and treatment. *Br J Anaesth* 2003; **91**(5): 718–29.

Question 6   Coeliac Plexus

Q	Marking guidance	Mark	Comments
a	Greater splanchnic nerve	1	*Sympathetic fibres from T5 to T9.*
	Lesser splanchnic nerve	1	*Sympathetic fibres from T10 to T11.*
	Least splanchnic nerve	1	*Sympathetic fibres from T12.*
			The coeliac plexus also receives parasympathetic input from the coeliac branch of the vagus nerve.
b	• Chronic pancreatitis • Malignancy of other upper abdominal organs: stomach, liver, gall bladder, duodenum, proximal small bowel	1 1	*The coeliac plexus provides sympathetic nervous supply from the lower oesophageal sphincter to the splenic flexure of the colon.*
c	• Neuropathic pain	1	*Neuropathic pain is caused by the tumour compressing nerves or invading the spinal cord.*
	• Somatic pain	1	*Somatic pain is caused by activation of pain receptors in either cutaneous or deep tissues, e.g. metastatic bone pain.*
d	**Preparation:** • AAGBI-recommended standard monitoring • Intravenous access • Resuscitation equipment available • Trained assistant • Stop before you block	6	Maximum of 2 marks for the block preparation. Maximum of 4 marks for the block-specific aspects.

(cont.)

Q	Marking guidance	Mark	Comments
	Block specific: • Prone position • X-ray screening (fluoroscopy) or CT guidance • Needle entry point: just below 12th rib • Advance needle until it hits L1 vertebral body • Withdraw needle and redirect to pass L1 vertebral body • Radio-opaque dye injected to confirm correct placement • Neurolytic agent injected		
e	Procedural complications: • Retroperitoneal haematoma • Intrathecal/epidural injection • Intravascular injection • Pneumothorax • Chylothorax • Visceral damage: kidneys/ ureters/upper abdominal organs • Infection • Paraplegia	Any 4	*The risk of intravascular injection is minimised by checking the needle position with radio-opaque dye before injection of alcohol/ phenol.* *Paraplegia may occur due to artery of Adamkiewicz spasm/trauma, spread of neurolytic to the spinal cord or hypotension.*
	Complications of sympathetic blockade: • Hypotension • Diarrhoea • Sexual dysfunction/impotence • Warm lower extremities	Any 3	

Suggested reading

J. Scott-Warren, A. Bhaskar. Cancer pain management: Part II: interventional techniques. *Cont Edu Anaesth Crit Care Pain* 2015; **15**(2): 68–72.

R. Menon, A. Swanepoel. Sympathetic blocks. *Cont Edu Anaesth Crit Care Pain* 2010; **10**(3): 88–92.

Question 7   Serotonin Syndrome

Q	Marking guidance	Mark	Comments
a	A potentially life-threatening condition associated with increased serotonergic activity in the central nervous system	1	*The main differential diagnosis is neuroleptic malignant syndrome, which is slower in onset and has a higher mortality. Dopamine agonism produces bradykinesia whereas serotonin agonism produces hyperkinesia.*
b	• Change in mental/cognitive status • Autonomic dysfunction • Neuromuscular excitability	3	*Mnemonic: 'Remember that patients CAN get serotonin syndrome' – Change in mental status (e.g. agitation, delirium), Autonomic dysfunction (e.g. sweating, hypertension, hyperthermia) and Neuromuscular excitability (e.g. myoclonus, tremor).*
c	Major criteria: • Recent addition or increase in a known serotinergic agent • No recent addition or increase of a neuroleptic agent • Absence of other possible aetiologies Minor criteria • Mental status changes (confusion, hypomania) • Agitation • Myoclonus • Hyperreflexia • Diaphoresis • Shivering • Tremor • Diarrhoea • Incoordination • Fever	Any 6	*Serotonin syndrome is a clinical diagnosis by means of the Sternbach diagnostic criteria – there are no confirmatory laboratory or radiological tests to confirm or refute diagnosis.* *The diagnosis can be made when all the major and three of the minor criteria are present.*

(cont.)

Q	Marking guidance	Mark	Comments
d	<u>Drugs that inhibit the reuptake/ metabolism of serotonin:</u> • Selective serotonin reuptake inhibitors (SSRIs) • Serotonin and noradrenaline reuptake inhibitors (SNRIs) • Opioids (tramadol/pethidine) • Monoamine oxidase inhibitors (MOAIs) • Tricyclic antidepressants <u>Drugs which stimulate serotonin release/serotonin agonists:</u> • Opioids (tramadol) • MDMA (ecstasy) • Amphetamines <u>Miscellaneous drugs:</u> • Lithium • Tryptophan	Any 4	
e	• Stop the offending agent • Critical care admission is indicated if there is severe hyperpyrexia, rhabdomyolysis, coagulopathy or acute respiratory distress syndrome • Control heart rate • Control blood pressure • Active cooling • Sedation for agitation • Renal support if rhabdomyolsis • Benzodiazepines for seizures • Specific treatments: oral cyproheptadine (an oral 5-HT2a antagonist)/intravenous chlorpromazine (but evidence is lacking)	4	*Serotonin syndrome typically resolves 24–72 hours after stopping the causative drug, although this does depend on the drug half-life and metabolites. The prognosis is generally good.*

(cont.)

Q	Marking guidance	Mark	Comments
f	Receptor subtypes: At least 14 (accept ≥ 12 subtypes) Receptor triggered: • 5-HT1a • 5-HT2	1 Any 1	

Suggested reading

J. Walsh. Serotonin syndrome. World Federation of Societies of Anaesthesiologists' Anaesthesia Tutorial of the Week 166. 2010. www.aagbi.org/sites/default/files/166-serotonin-syndrome.pdf. (Accessed 28 October 2018).

S. Chinniah, J. L. H. French, D. M. Levy. Serotonin and anaesthesia. *Cont Edu Anaesth Crit Care Pain* 2008; **8**(2): 43–5.

Question 8 Chemotherapy

Q	Marking guidance	Mark	Comments
a	• Improve chance of complete resection and survival • Reduce need for more complex or disfiguring surgery	Any 1	*Patients commonly receive neo-adjuvant chemotherapy for the following cancers: breast, oesophageal, gastric, bowel, ovarian, germ cell and osteosarcoma.*
b	• Alkylating agents • Anti-metabolites • Topoisomerase interactive agents • Anti-microtubule agents • Hormonal agents • Tyrosine kinase inhibitors/ antibody agents	Any 3	*E.g. cyclophosphamide, cisplatin* *E.g. methotrexate, 5-fluorouracil* *E.g. irinotecan, doxorubicin, bleomycin* *E.g. paclitaxel* *E.g. anastrazole, luteinising hormone-releasing hormone analogues* *E.g. trastuzumab*
c	<u>Cardiac:</u> • Hypotension/hypertension • Arrhythmias • Myocardial infarction • Congestive cardiac failure • Cardiomyopathy • Myocarditis/pericarditis <u>Respiratory:</u> • Pneumonitis • Pulmonary embolism • Acute pneumonia <u>Gastrointestinal:</u> • Dehydration/electrolyte disturbance from nausea/ vomiting • Mucositis <u>Hepatic:</u> • Cholestasis • Hepatocellular necrosis • Hepatic cirrhosis/fibrosis	Any 2 Any 2 2 Any 2	*Pre-operative assessment should include a focussed history of cancer management.* *A drug history, including the precise chemotherapy regime used and any specific toxic effects suffered by the patient, should be sought.* *Clinical features of toxicity which may alert you to more serious systemic complications include shortness of breath, palpitations, chest pain and fever.* *Clinical examination may also reveal signs that require further*

Q	Marking guidance	Mark	Comments
	Haemopoietic: • Anaemia • Thrombocytopenia • Neutropenia (accept 'myelosuppression' or 'pancytopenia' for 1 mark)	Any 2	*investigation before surgery.* *Routine investigations should include full blood count, biochemistry and an ECG.*
	Central nervous system: • Peripheral neuropathy • Seizures • Encephalopathy • Vocal cord palsy • Autonomic neuropathy Do NOT accept 'neuropathy' – must be specific	Any 2	*Other investigations, e.g. chest X-ray, arterial blood gas, pulmonary function tests and echocardiography, may be required, depending upon the treatment regimen used.*
d	• Oxygen therapy should be avoided if at all possible • Utilise the lowest inspired oxygen fraction possible • If patient is hypoxic, oxygen therapy should be minimised to maintain saturations of 88%–92% • High oxygen concentrations should only be used for immediate life-saving indications	Any 3	*Bleomycin is often used to treat germ cell tumours and Hodgkin's disease.* *Bleomycin therapy has the potential to cause subacute pulmonary damage that can progress to life-threatening pulmonary fibrosis. This is a lifelong risk.* *Pulmonary toxicity occurs in 6%–10% of patients and can be fatal.* *Exposure to high-inspired concentration oxygen therapy, even for short periods, is implicated in triggering a rapidly progressive pulmonary toxicity in patients previously treated with bleomycin.*

(cont.)

Q	Marking guidance	Mark	Comments
e	Vincristine	1	*The vinca alkaloid vincristine can cause severe neurotoxicity. It is often used to treat lymphoma and leukaemia.*

Suggested reading

N. Allen, C. Siller, A. Breen. Anaesthetic implications of chemotherapy. *Cont Edu Anaesth Crit Care Pain* 2012; **12**(2): 52–6.

Question 9 Trauma and Splenectomy

Q	Marking guidance	Mark	Comments
a	• Primary trauma survey • Cervical spine immobilisation • Wide-bore intravenous access • Group O negative blood • Send blood samples to the laboratory • Cross-match blood • Permissive hypotension • Oxygen therapy (target saturations > 95%) • Activate major haemorrhage protocol • Analgesia • Assess neurovascular status of left lower limb • Patient warming • Intravenous tranexamic acid • Orthopaedic review • General surgical review Not acceptable: ABCDE assessment (not specific enough)	Any 6	*This patient's observations suggest severe haemorrhagic shock and likely require resuscitation with blood products (not crystalloid). Blood samples should be sent to the laboratory as soon as possible.*
b	• Focussed Abdominal with Sonography in Trauma (FAST) scan → hypoechoic rim around spleen; fluid in Morrison's pouch (hepatorenal space) • CT abdominal scan → haemoperitoneum; hypodense areas in spleen represent parenchymal disruption; contrast blush or extravasation	1 1 1 1	

(cont.)

Q	Marking guidance	Mark	Comments
c	Immunological: • Storage of lymphocytes	Any 3	*Up to a quarter of the body's lymphocytes can be stored in the spleen.*
	• Innate immune response: removal of blood-borne pathogens by macrophages in red pulp • Adaptive immune response: white pulp contains separate areas for B and T cells		
	Non-immunological: • Removal of old red blood cells • Spleen acts as a blood reservoir (250 mL) • Store of platelets • Removal of old platelets	Any 2	
d	• Pneumococcal vaccine • *Haemophilus influenzae* type B • Meningococcal C Timing: 2 weeks after traumatic splenectomy	4	*The spleen is essential for protection against encapsulated bacteria.*
e	Penicillin V	1	*Or clarithromycin if penicillin allergic.*

Suggested reading

L. Gent, P. Blackie. The spleen. *BJA Educ* 2017; **17**(6): 214–20.

Question 10   Parkinson's Disease

Q	Marking guidance	Mark	Comments
a	• Bradykinesia • Muscle rigidity • Asymmetric resting tremor	1 1 1	
b	Constitutional: • Fatigue • Depression/anxiety • Sleep disturbance • Constipation	Any 1	
	Motor symptoms: • Gait change • Dysphagia • Micrographia • Soft speech • Postural instability	Any 1	
	Neuropsychiatric symptoms: • Cognitive disturbance (inattention, slowed cognitive speed, poor problem solving) • Dementia	Any 1	*Dementia is common in advanced Parkinson's disease: >80% after 20 years.*
	Autonomic symptoms: • Postural hypotension • Sialorrhoea • Urinary dysfunction • Sexual dysfunction	Any 1	*Sialorrhoea (drooling) is seen in advanced Parkinson's and may simply be a result of impaired swallowing.*
c	• Loss of dopaminergic neurons • From the pars compacta region of the substantia nigra	1 1	
d	• Dopamine precursors, e.g. levodopa • Dopamine agonists: e.g. pramipexole, ropinirole, rotigotine, apomorphine • Monoamine oxidase B inhibitors (MAOIBs), e.g. selegiline • Catechol-O-methyl transferase inhibitors (COMTIs), e.g. entacapone • Glutamate antagonist, e.g. amantadine	Any 3	No half marks – must have a correct class with corresponding drug name to gain the whole mark.

(cont.)

Q	Marking guidance	Mark	Comments
e	• Apomorphine (subcutaneously administered dopamine agonist)	1	
	Advantage: can be used in advanced Parkinson's disease	1	
	Disadvantage: highly emetogenic, risk of severe hypotension	1	
	• Rotigotine (transdermal dopamine agonist)	1	
	Advantage: ease of use	1	
	Disadvantage: not sufficiently potent to manage patients on higher-dose antiparkinsonian drug regimes	1	
f	• Domperidone • Ondansetron • Cyclizine	Any 2	*Many commonly used antiemetics are contra-indicated in Parkinson's disease, e.g. prochlorperazine, metoclopramide.*

Suggested reading

D. J. Chambers, J. Sebastian, D. J. Ahearn. Parkinson's disease. *BJA Educ* 2017; **17**(4): 145–9.

Question 11 Carbon Dioxide Measurement

Q	Marking guidance	Mark	Comments
a	• Capnometry: measurement/ analysis of CO_2 in a sample of gas	1	*Although the terms are sometimes used synonymously, capnometry refers to measurement and may give a numerical display. Capnography is the continuous measurement and waveform display (capnogram).*
	• Capnography: continuous monitoring of the concentration or partial pressure of CO_2	1	
b	• Molecules containing dissimilar atoms absorb infrared radiation	1	*The generated infrared radiation is focussed through a chopper wheel which has a number of filters to select specific wavelengths. A reference channel is positioned alongside the sample channel.*
	• Molecules absorb infrared radiation of specific wavelengths	1	
	• Absorption is proportional to the concentration of the attenuating molecules in the sample (Beer's law)	1	
c	• Photoacoustic spectroscopy • Piezoelectric absorption • Refractometry • Raman scattering • Mass spectrometry	5	*Infra-red spectroscopy is a more compact and relatively cheap method. CO_2 absorbs infra-red light at 4.3 μm.*
d	• Phase two: both dead space AND alveolar gas expired	1	*If alveoli contained the same partial pressure of CO_2, phase three would be a straight line. However, alveoli with lower $\dot{V}/\dot{Q}$ ratios/longer time constants contribute to the slight upward slope seen.*
	• Phase three: alveolar gas expired	1	
	End-tidal CO_2 is determined at the end of phase three – see diagram	1	

(cont.)

Q	Marking guidance	Mark	Comments
e	• Confirmation of airway placement and patency • Monitoring ventilation rate • Assessing adequacy of chest compressions • Identifying ROSC	4	*Waveform capnography during cardiopulmonary resuscitation has been incorporated into resuscitation guidance. End-tidal CO_2 may be used to prognosticate, but only as part of a wider multi-modal approach.*
f	• CO_2 diffuses across semi-permeable/rubber/Teflon membrane • Dissociates into hydrogen ions • Hydrogen ions are produced in proportion to the PCO_2 • Measured by pH electrode/potential difference generated between sample and buffer solution	Any 3	*The Severinghaus electrode is a modified pH electrode. If a glass membrane separates two solutions of different hydrogen ion concentration, a potential difference proportional to the ion gradient develops which can then be measured.*

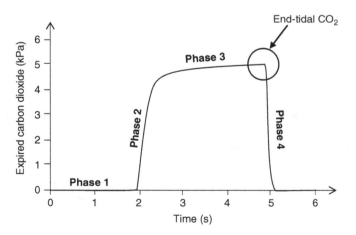

Figure 5.11d Answer

Suggested reading

I. Kerslake, F. Kelly. Uses of capnography in the critical care unit. *BJA Educ* 2017; **17**(5): 178–83.

Q	Marking guidance	Mark	Comments
a	Sensitivity refers to the ability of the clinical test to correctly identify those patients with a difficult airway $\text{Sensitivity} = \dfrac{\text{True positives}}{\text{True positves} + \text{false negatives}}$	1 2	Two marks for correct formula
b	Specificity refers to the ability of the clinical test to correctly identify those patients without a difficult airway $\text{Specificity} = \dfrac{\text{True negatives}}{\text{True negatives} + \text{false positives}}$	1 2	Two marks for correct formula
c	Meta-analysis = statistical discipline of assimilating data from multiple similar studies	1	*A meta-analysis is a quantitative form of systematic review.*
	To measure an overall effect using all of the available evidence	1	
d	Forest plot = graphical means of comparing studies included in a meta-analysis	1	
	Square: Each study is represented by a square (whose size represents the study size)	1	
	and a line (which represents the 95% confidence interval)	1	
	Diamond: The diamond at the bottom of the Forest plot represents the pooled data from all studies;	1	
	its width represents the 95% confidence interval	1	
e	• Publication bias	Any 2	*Studies with positive or statistically significant results are more likely to be published in scientific journals.*
	• Replication bias		*Data may be replicated in a meta-analysis if they have been used in multiple studies.*
	• Language bias		*If only studies published in English are included, the data may be incomplete.*

(cont.)

Q	Marking guidance	Mark	Comments
f	1. (highest level) Systematic review of multiple randomised controlled trials; randomised controlled trial 2. Cohort study 3. Case–control study 4. Case series 5. (lowest level) Case report; expert opinion	5	

Suggested reading

A. G. Lalkhen, A. McCluskey. Statistics V: Introduction to clinical trials and systematic reviews. *Cont Edu Anaesth Crit Care Pain* 2008; **8**(4): 143–6.

A. G. Lalkhen, A. McCluskey. Clinical tests: sensitivity and specificity. *Cont Edu Anaesth Crit Care Pain* 2008; **8**(6): 221–3.

Paper 6 Answers

Question 1 Acoustic Neuroma

Q	Marking guidance	Mark	Comments
a	• Unilateral sensorineural hearing loss • Unilateral tinnitus • Balance problems/vertigo • Cranial nerve V (trigeminal) palsy causing facial numbness/paraesthesia, decreased corneal reflex	4	*NB Cranial nerve VII (facial) palsy is rare but is a complication of surgical excision. Headache is uncommon, except for large tumours.* *Acoustic neuroma is a benign tumour of the Schwann cells of the vestibular division of the eighth cranial nerve. Patients usually present with symptoms when the tumour is relatively small.*
b	• Unilateral weakness of facial muscles • Unilateral loss of taste/metallic taste • Unilateral decrease in salivation • Unilateral decrease in tear production • Inability to close eye/ptosis	Any 4	 *Chorda tympani damage.* *Greater petrosal nerve palsy.* *Greater petrosal nerve palsy.* *Damage to temporal and zygomatic branches.*
c	• Prone • Lateral/park bench • Sitting	Any 2	*The sitting position offers the best surgical operating conditions, but carries a high risk of venous air embolism.*

(cont.)

Q	Marking guidance	Mark	Comments
d	• Padding of elbows/supination of forearm: risk of ulnar nerve compression injury • Padding of heels • Careful securing of endotracheal tube, so as to not cause pressure on lips • Avoid straight legs: pillow under knees • Avoid extreme head rotation: risk of brachial plexus stretch injury • Avoid tension on urinary catheter: pressure injury to bladder neck • Tape eyelids closed; padding of eyes	Any 4	
e	• Use of opioid to suppress cough reflex • Spontaneous breathing deep extubation • Exchange endotracheal tube for laryngeal mask airway • Lignocaine (intravenous bolus or within endotracheal cuff)	Any 3	*Most commonly achieved through use of a remifentanil infusion.*
f	• Haematoma: subdural/extradural/intraparenchymal • Direct injury to brainstem during surgery • Hydrocephalus	3	*The posterior fossa is a very small space: a small volume of blood or parenchymal oedema can compress the brainstem or obstruct cerebrospinal flow.*

Suggested reading

S. Jagannathan, H. Krovvidi. Anaesthetic considerations for posterior fossa surgery. *Cont Edu Anaesth Crit Care Pain* 2014; **14**(5): 202–6.

Question 2 Heart Failure

Q	Marking guidance	Mark	Comments
a	• Hypertension • Diabetes mellitus • Ischaemic heart disease • Valvular disease • Cardiomyopathies • Alcohol abuse	Any 3	*Mechanisms of heart failure can be subdivided into three types:* • *Myocyte death (e.g. ischaemic heart disease, alcohol, myocarditis)* • *Myocyte dysfunction (e.g. pregnancy, nutritional deficiencies)* • *Circulatory dysfunction (e.g. valvular heart disease, protracted severe anaemia)*
b	• Hypertrophy • Dilatation	1 1	*As myocardial contractility decreases, the stroke volume (SV) decreases, which leads to an increase in left ventricular end-diastolic pressure (LVEDP). According to the Frank–Starling mechanism, this increased LVEDP restores SV. In the longer term, this left ventricular volume overload causes myocardial re-modelling – the subsequent hypertrophy and dilatation result in an increase in ventricular wall stress and oxygen demand.*
c	See diagram	6	*Compared to the normal cardiac loop, the failing left ventricular loop demonstrates* • *rightward shift of end-systolic volume, due to impaired contractility* • *raised LVEDP due to impaired myocardial relaxation*

(cont.)

Q	Marking guidance	Mark	Comments
			• *a reduction in the width (i.e. reduction in SV) as a consequence of a higher end-systolic volume* • *a lower end-diastolic volume.*
d	• Renin–angiotensin–aldosterone system (RAAS) • Sympathetic nervous system (SNS)	1 1	*The reduction in cardiac output (CO) activates the RAAS, resulting in salt and water retention and an increase in circulating volume. Although this would normally restore CO according to the Frank–Starling mechanism, the result in the failing heart is volume overload and increased systemic vascular resistance.* *Activation of the SNS would normally restore CO through an increase in heart rate and contractility. However, in the failing heart, increased heart rate impairs filling and increases myocardial work and oxidative stress, risking sub-endocardial ischaemia.*
e	• Angiotensin II receptor blocker OR angiotensin-converting enzyme inhibitor • Neprilysin inhibitor (Sacubitril) • β-blockade • Diuretics	Any 3	*Neprilysin is an endopeptidase which metabolises brain natriuretic peptide (BNP), released by the cardiac ventricles in volume overload. Sacubitril inhibits neprilysin, thus increasing BNP which then acts to promote natriuresis.*

Q	Marking guidance	Mark	Comments
f	• Maintenance of preload/high central venous pressure (CVP)	Any 4	*High CVP to facilitate filling of poorly compliant ventricle.*
	• Avoid tachycardia		*To preserve diastolic time.*
	• Avoid/promptly treat arrhythmia		*Ensure atrial kick to fill against high LVEDP.*
	• Maintain contractility/positive inotropy		*May require positive inotropes to achieve this.*
	• Avoid acute increases in afterload		

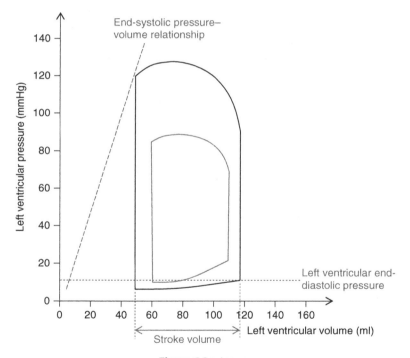

Figure 6.2c Answer

Suggested reading

A. Kotze, S. Howell. Heart failure: pathophysiology, risk assessment, community management and anaesthesia. *Cont Edu Anaesth Crit Care Pain.* 2008; **8**(5): 161–6.

Question 3 Acute Asthma

Q	Marking guidance	Mark	Comments
a	• Oxygen titrated to saturation • Salbutamol 5 mg nebulised • Ipratropium 0.5 mg nebulised • Hydrocortisone 200 mg/ prednisolone 40 mg • Magnesium 2 g intravenous	Any 4	*According to the British Thoracic Society (BTS) guidelines. Nebulisers should be driven by oxygen.*
b	• Peak expiratory flow rate (PEFR) 33% best of predicted • $SpO_2 > 92\%$ • $P_aO_2 > 8$ kPa • Normal P_aCO_2 (4.6–6.0 kPa) • Silent chest • Cyanosis • Feeble respiratory effort • Bradycardia • Arrhythmia • Hypotension • Exhaustion • Confusion	Any 6	*According to the BTS guidelines, a diagnosis of life-threatening asthma may be made if the patient has any ONE of these symptoms.* *Diagnostic criteria of 'near fatal' asthma in adults are a raised P_aCO_2 and/or requiring mechanical ventilation with raised inflation pressures.*
c	<u>Absolute indications:</u> • Coma • Respiratory arrest • Cardiac arrest • Severe refractory hypoxaemia	4	
	<u>Relative indications include:</u> • Poor response to initial management • Fatigue • Somnolence • Cardiovascular compromise	Any 4	

(cont.)

Q	Marking guidance	Mark	Comments
	• Development of a pneumothorax		
d	• Respiratory rate: 12–14 breaths/min → prevent gas trapping and hyperinflation • PEEP: ≤5 cmH$_2$0 → as intrinsic PEEP is high in acute asthma, the extrinsic PEEP should be low • I:E ratio: up to 1:4 → to allow adequate expiration and prevent gas trapping • P max: <35 cmH$_2$0 → to prevent barotrauma (especially pneumothorax)	4	*The aim is to allow oxygenation and break bronchospasm whilst preventing complications of high-pressure ventilation (e.g. acute lung injury/ barotrauma).*
e	• Inhaled anaesthetic agent (e.g. sevoflurane) • Intravenous ketamine	2	Not acceptable: magnesium – this should have been given prior to intubation.

Suggested reading

D. Stanley, W. Tunnicliffe. Management of life-threatening asthma in adults. *Cont Edu Anaesth Crit Care Pain* 2008; **8**(3); 95–9.

British Thoracic Society and Scottish Intercollegiate Guidelines Network. British guideline on the management of asthma. 2016. www.brit-thoracic.org.uk/document-library/clinical-information/asthma/btssign-asthma-guideline-quick-reference-guide-2016. (Accessed 7 October 2018).

Question 4   Inhaled Foreign Body

Q	Marking guidance	Mark	Comments
a	Inhaled foreign body/foreign body aspiration	1	*Foreign body (FB) aspiration most commonly occurs in 1- to 3-year-olds (boys > girls). Children of this age are prone to FB aspiration because they* • *Put objects in their mouths* • *Have less ability to chew food*
b	• Tracheal tug/intercostal and subcostal recession • Use of accessory muscles/tripod position • Seesaw pattern/paradoxical abdominal breathing • Tachycardia/sweating • Peripheral/central cyanosis • Nasal flaring • Grunting/stridor	Any 4	
c	• Nil apparent • Aspirated radio-opaque object (must specify 'radio-opaque') • Pneumothorax • Consolidation • Collapse • Hyperinflation/gas trapping • Mediastinal shift	Any 4	*The majority of inhaled material is organic in origin and therefore a chest X-ray may fail to demonstrate an abnormality, especially in the first 24 hours.* *The absence of radiographic abnormalities does not exclude the diagnosis of an inhaled FB.*

Q	Marking guidance	Mark	Comments
d	Advantages: • Avoids need for awake cannulation • Allows for pre-oxygenation • Reduced risk of distal movement of FB • Lessens degree of distal air-trapping • Allows rapid assessment of ventilation post-retrieval	Any 3	*The alternative technique would be IV induction and positive pressure ventilation.* *The advantages of this include:* • *Reduced aspiration risk* • *Reduced risk of coughing* • *Reduced atelectasis*
	Disadvantages: • Difficulty maintaining depth of anaesthesia • Required depth of anaesthesia to eliminate airway reflexes may cause $\dot{V}/\dot{Q}$ mismatch and cardiovascular compromise • Risk of coughing/patient movement • Risk of hypercapnia due to resistance once scope inserted • Harder to manage any IV maintenance therapy as need to maintain spontaneous respiratory effort	Any 3	• *Optimal oxygenation and ventilation prior to bronchoscopy* • *Easier to use IV maintenance as airway and ventilation already controlled* *Disadvantages include:* • *Necessitates awake cannulation* • *May move FB distally* • *Unable to assess ventilation post-procedure until cessation of paralysis and anaesthesia* • *May increase distal air-trapping*
e	Drug: Lignocaine Dose: 4 mg/kg (accept 2–4 mg/kg)	1 1	*The maximum recommended dose of lignocaine (without adrenaline) is usually quoted as 3 mg/kg. For airway topicalisation, this may be increased to 4 mg/kg in children as much of the lignocaine is ultimately swallowed.*

(cont.)

Q	Marking guidance	Mark	Comments
f	• Infection/abscess • Laryngeal oedema/stridor • Pneumothorax/haemothorax • Respiratory failure/ongoing O_2 requirement	Any 3	

Suggested reading

A. Skinner. Inhaled foreign body in children. World Federation of Societies of Anaesthesiologists' Anaesthesia Tutorial of the Week 99. 2008. www.aagbi.org/sites/default/files/99-Inhaled-foreign-body-in-children.pdf. (Accessed 16 September 2018).

Question 5 Post-partum Haemorrhage (PPH)

Q	Marking guidance	Mark	Comments
a	• Uterine atony (not acceptable: 'tone')	1	*Primary postpartum haemorrhage (PPH) is defined as loss of > 500 mL from the genital tract within 24 hours of delivery.*
	• Retained products of conception (not acceptable: 'tissue')	1	
	• Genital tract trauma	1	
	• Coagulopathy (not acceptable: 'thrombin')	1	*A mnemonic for the common causes of PPH is the '4 Ts' – Tone, Tissue, Trauma, Thrombin.*
b	• Syntocinon intravenous 5 IU		*Hyperthermia and diarrhoea may be seen following administration of misoprostol.*
	• Tranexamic acid intravenous 1 g	1	
	• Carboprost intramuscular 250 µg	2	
	• Misoprostol per rectum 800 µg (accept 600 µg to 1 mg)	2	
	• Ergometrine intramuscular 500 µg (accept intravenous, accept 250 µg)	2	*Ergometrine should be avoided in patients with pre-eclampsia as it can exacerbate hypertension.*
	Units must be present to gain marks		
c	• Bimanual compression/uterine massage	Any 6	*Resuscitative measures should be taken alongside those to stop the bleeding.*
	• Uterine balloon tamponade/Bakri balloon/Rusche balloon		
	• B-Lynch suture		*The key to successful management is early senior input. Think ahead and act early.*
	• Interventional radiology		
	• Vessel ligation (internal iliac, uterine, hypogastric, ovarian)		
	• Hysterectomy		
	• Aortic compression		
d	Asthma	1	*Risk of bronchospasm.*
e	• Puerperal sepsis (accept: infection)	1	*Endometritis is a common cause of postnatal morbidity.*
	• Retained products of conception	1	

Suggested reading

F. Plaat, A. Shonfeld. Major obstetric haemorrhage. *BJA Educ* 2015; **15**(4): 190–3.

Royal College of Obstetrician and Gynaecologists. Green-top Guideline No.52: Prevention and Management of Postpartum Haemorrhage. 2006. www.rcog.org.uk/en/ guidelines-research-services/guidelines/ gtg52. (Accessed 13 October 2018).

Question 6 Phantom Limb Pain

Q	Marking guidance	Mark	Comments
a	Equipment or drug delivery issue: • PCA empty/malfunctioned • IV cannula tissued Acute surgical complication: • Bleeding • Haematoma • Infection Others: • Wearing off of oral co-analgesia/ local anaesthesia/regional anaesthesia • Stump pain: common in early post-operative period	Any 4	*Phantom limb pain usually occurs within the first week following amputation. The pain feels as if it is located in a distal part of amputated limb, and is often burning/shooting in nature.* *Stump pain is an acute nociceptive pain which usually resolves as the wound heals.*
b	• Take a pain history and examine patient • Review drug prescription: ensure any regular analgesia due has been given • Check PCA pump is working correctly, review PCA chart and ensure that cannula is patent • Surgical review to exclude complications such as bleeding or infection	Any 3	
c	• For neuropathic pain: amitriptyline or gabapentinoids • Intravenous ketamine • Intravenous lignocaine/ lignocaine patch over stump • Indwelling peripheral nerve catheter	Any 3	*If the cause is phantom limb pain, this is often resistant to systemic opioids.*
d	Up to 80% (accept 70%–90%)	1	
e	• Pre-amputation pain • Presence of stump pain • Bilateral limb amputations • Lower limb amputations	Any 3	

(cont.)

Q	Marking guidance	Mark	Comments
	• Repeated limb surgeries • Increasing age		
f	Peripheral causes: • Spontaneous discharge of afferent neurons • Spontaneous discharge in the dorsal root ganglia • Upregulation of sodium channels • Coupling to the sympathetic nervous system • Neuromas	3	*The exact mechanism for the development of PLP is likely to be multi-faceted, with peripheral, spinal cord and central contributions.*
	Spinal cord causes: • Re-organisation of c-fibres at lamina • Sensitisation of dorsal horn	2	
	Central cause: • Cortical re-organisation	1	

Suggested reading

M. J. E. Neil. Pain after amputation
BJA Educ 2016; **16**(3): 107–12.

Question 7 Sickle Cell Disease

Q	Marking guidance	Mark	Comments
a	• Haemoglobin electrophoresis • Sickledex test • Peripheral blood film	Any 2	*Sickledex test will detect levels of HbS > 10%, but cannot distinguish between SCD and sickle cell trait. Blood film may reveal sickled red cells, or a raised reticulocyte count.*
b	<u>Mendelian inheritance:</u> Autosomal recessive <u>Genetics:</u> • Amino acid substitution: glutamic acid for valine • At the sixth position of the haemoglobin β chain • On chromosome 11	1 Any 2	
c	• Hypoxaemia • Acidosis • Dehydration • Hypothermia • Infection • Strenuous exercise • Venous stasis	Any 5	*Alcohol intake may cause dehydration.* *This may cause lactic acidosis.* *Tourniquets are traditionally avoided for this reason.*
d	• Small vessel occlusion • Haemolytic anaemia/greatly reduced half-life of RBCs	1 1	*The half-life of a RBC decreases from 120 days to just 12 days.*

(cont.)

Q	Marking guidance	Mark	Comments
e	• Haemolytic anaemia	Any 8	
	• Occlusive crises, e.g. dactylitis		*Abdominal pain due to vessel occlusion may be difficult to distinguish from other causes of acute abdomen.*
	• Acute chest syndrome		*Defined as a temperature ≥ 38.5°C, chest pain or respiratory distress and new lobar infiltrates on chest X-ray.*
	• Stroke		
	• Aplastic crisis		*Usually precipitated by parvovirus B19 infection.*
	• Acute splenic sequestration		*Large numbers of RBCs are sequestered in the spleen, causing a sudden drop in haemoglobin and cardiovascular collapse.*
	• Splenic infarction		*Caused by repeated sickling episodes, makes patients susceptible to encapsulated bacteria.*
	• Osteomyelitis		*Most common pathogens: salmonella and staphylococci.*
	• Priapism		
	• Avascular necrosis		*Most often of the femoral head.*
	• Gallstones		*Due to haemolytic anaemia.*
	• Sickle retinopathy		
	• Leg ulcers		
	• Chronic renal failure		

Suggested reading

M. Wilson, P. Forsyth, J. Whiteside. Haemoglobinopathy and sickle cell disease. *BJA Educ* 2010; **10**(1): 24–8.

C. Locke. Anaesthetic management of sickle cell disease in children. World Federation of Societies of Anaesthesiologists' Anaesthesia Tutorial of the Week **153**. 2009. www.aagbi .org/sites/default/files/153-Sickle-cell-dis ease-in-children.pdf. (Accessed 13 September 2018).

Question 8 Local Anaesthetic Toxicity

Q	Marking guidance	Mark	Comments
a	• Frequent aspiration • Incremental injection • Test dose • Maintain verbal contact with patient • Use of 'tracer', e.g. adrenaline	Any 4	*Although these steps are often suggested, there is little evidence to suggest they reduce the risk of LA toxicity.*
b	• Lower a_1-acid glycoprotein levels (accept lower protein binding) • Increased vascularity of epidural space • Results in high peak free LA concentrations	1 1 1	*Lower protein binding and rapid absorption of LA increases the risk of toxicity in pregnancy.*
c	(Both components must be correct to score each mark). Lignocaine: 3 mg/kg without, 7 mg/kg with Bupivacaine 2 mg/kg without, 2 mg/kg with Ropivacaine 3 mg/kg without, 3 mg/kg with Prilocaine 6 mg/kg	 1 1 1 1	*Fixed dosing rules do not account for the wider clinical context; the epidural route carries a greater risk of LA toxicity than subcutaneous injection.*
d	• Renal failure • Liver failure • Cardiac failure • Elderly patients • Paediatric patients	Any 4	*LA clearance is reduced in renal impairment and liver disease. Patients with cardiac failure are more susceptible to myocardial depression and arrhythmias.*
e	Concentration: 20% Bolus dose: 105 mL (accept 100 mL) Initial infusion rate: 1050 mL/h (accept 1000 mL/h) Maximum dose: 840 mL	1 1 1 1	*Initial bolus is 1.5 mL/kg followed by an infusion of 15 mL/kg/h. Two further bolus doses can be given at 5 min intervals, with the rate of infusion doubled to 30 mL/kg/h if the clinical situation is unchanged.*

(cont.)

Q	Marking guidance	Mark	Comments
f	Continue cardiopulmonary resuscitation for > 1 hour	1	

Suggested reading

L. E. Christie, J. Picard, G. L. Weinberg.
Local anaesthetic systemic toxicity.
BJA Educ 2015; **15**(3): 136–42.

Question 9   Renal Transplant

Q	Marking guidance	Mark	Comments
a	• Diabetes mellitus (25%) • Glomerulonephritis (14%) • Hypertension (8%) • Polycystic kidney disease (8%) • Pyelonephritis (7%) • Renal vascular disease (5%)	Any 4	*The remaining 33% of cases are described as 'other (18%)' and 'uncertain aetiology (15%)', according to the UK Renal Registry.*
b	History: • Aetiology of ESRF • Symptoms consistent with ischaemic heart disease (IHD) • Dry weight/any fluid restriction/whether the patient is anuric • Timing of dialysis – is further dialysis required pre-operatively? • Current medication • Assessment of reflux/delayed gastric emptying, may require rapid sequence induction	Any 3	*ESRF is an independent risk factor for IHD.* *May be caused by autonomic neuropathy if aetiology of ESRF is diabetes mellitus.*
	Clinical examination: • Assessment of current fluid status • Status of fistula site • Assessment of venous access	Any 2	 *Hands are preferred, in case subsequent arterio-venous fistulae are required.*
	Pre-operative investigations: • ECG • Haemoglobin • White cell count • Pre-operative chest X-ray • Post-dialysis electrolytes • Post-dialysis acid–base status • Blood pressure	Any 3	 *Patients with renal failure are often anaemic.* *Infection (e.g. urinary tract, dialysis line) and subsequent immunosuppression may result in overwhelming sepsis.* *To correlate with clinical assessment of fluid status.* *Bloods are taken routinely before and after a dialysis session.*

(cont.)

Q	Marking guidance	Mark	Comments
c	• Avoid cannulating the limb • Wrapping and padding the limb • Not using non-invasive blood pressure on the same limb	Any 2	
d	Blood pressure management: • Mean arterial pressure ≥ 90 mmHg • Normotension especially at the time of cross-clamp removal Fluid management: • <2500 mL crystalloid/colloid • Fluid loading to optimise cardiac output • Aim for CVP 12–14 mmHg • Mannitol	Any 3	*Adjusted upwards for untreated hypertensive patients.* Maximum of 2 marks for fluid management *Mannitol is used as a colloid, and as a free-radical scavenger, but there is little evidence of improved graft survival.*
e	Analgesic options: • Morphine PCA at reduced dose of 0.5 mg bolus (must say reduced dose for mark) • Fentanyl PCA • Regional technique such as transverse abdominis plane (TAP) block • Neuraxial blockade Analgesic to avoid: Non-steroidal anti-inflammatories (NSAIDs)	Any 2 1	*Renal function may improve only slowly after the transplant. Fentanyl is preferred over morphine in renal failure.* *There is an increased risk of spinal haematoma in ESRF patients. Epidural analgesia may risk post-operative hypotension. NSAIDs reduce renal blood flow, may threaten the transplanted kidney and exacerbate renal cyclosporin toxicity.*

Suggested reading

D. Mayhew, D. Ridgway, J. M. Hunter.
Update on the intraoperative
management of adult cadaveric
renal transplantation. *BJA Educ*
2016; **16**(2): 53–7.

Question 10 Hypertension

Q	Marking guidance	Mark	Comments
a	Aortic arch Carotid sinus (accept carotid body) (must have both correct answers to score 1 mark)	1	*Aortic arch baroreceptors are innervated by the vagus nerve, whilst carotid sinus baroreceptors are innervated by the glossopharyngeal nerve.*
b	Increase in blood pressure (BP) sensed by high-pressure baroreceptors → Increased action potentials transmitted along vagus and glossopharyngeal nerves to nucleus tractus solitarius (accept medulla oblongata) → Inhibition of vasomotor area → Reduced sympathetic outflow → bradycardia and vasodilatation	Any 3	*Regulation over subsequent minutes to hours is via low-pressure receptors in the atria and great veins, resulting in anti-diuretic hormone (ADH), brain/atrial natriuretic factor (BNP/ANP) and renin release. Long-term BP control is through the renin–angiotensin–aldosterone system (RAAS).*
c	Definitions: (must have both correct for 1 mark) • Primary: hypertension with no single known cause • Secondary: hypertension with an identifiable organic cause	1	4 marks overall for causes; maximum 2 marks from renal, endocrine and other classes. *Approximately 5% of hypertensive patients have secondary hypertension.*
	Renal causes: • Diabetic nephropathy • Polycystic kidney disease • Glomerular disease • Renovascular hypertension	Max 2	
	Endocrine causes: • Cushing's syndrome • Conn's syndrome • Hypo- and hyperthyroidism • Hyperparathyroidism • Phaeochromocytoma	Max 2	
	Others: • Sleep apnoea • Coarctation of the aorta • Pregnancy	Max 2	

(cont.)

Q	Marking guidance	Mark	Comments
d	Cardiac: • Left ventricular hypertrophy • Diastolic dysfunction • Heart failure • Atherosclerotic coronary artery disease	Any 2	*Other complications of untreated hypertension: hypertensive retinopathy, peripheral vascular disease.*
	Renal: • Glomerular injury • Glomerulosclerosis • Renal tubular ischaemia • End-stage renal failure	Any 2	
	Cerebrovascular: • Cerebrovascular accident • Impaired cognition • Hypertensive encephalopathy	Any 2	
e	Repeat the reading in a quiet environment ensuring that the correct technique is used	1	
f	>180/110 mmHg	1	*Recent studies suggest that patients with moderate hypertension have only a small increase in perioperative risk when compared to patients with severe hypertension.*
g	Blood pressure goal: Avoid > 20% reduction in systolic blood pressure	1	
	Reason: Organ autoregulation will be shifted to higher blood pressure	1	
h	Silent myocardial ischaemia (accept perioperative cardiac event)	1	*Silent myocardial infarction may be missed without continuous ECG monitoring or serial serum troponin measurements.*

Suggested reading

V. Nadella, S. J. Howell. Hypertension: pathophysiology and perioperative implications. *Cont Edu Anaesth Crit Care Pain* 2015; **15**(6): 275–9.

A. Hartle, T. McCormack, J. Carlisle, et al. The measurement of adult blood pressure and management of hypertension before elective surgery. *Anaesthesia* 2016; **71**(3): 326–37.

Question 11 Carotid Endarterectomy

Q	Marking guidance	Mark	Comments
a	70%–99% stenosis (accept ≥ 70%)	1	*Based on the North American Symptomatic Endarterectomy Trial (NASCET) and the European Carotid Surgery Trial (ECST).*
b	Where carotid stenosis meets the criteria in part (a), the patient should undergo CEA within a maximum of 2 weeks from the onset of TIA symptoms	1	*National Institute for Health and Care Excellence Clinical Guideline 68.*
c	Advantages: • Allows direct real-time neurological monitoring • Avoids the risk of airway intervention: intubation and extubation • Reduced shunt rate • Reduced length of hospital stay • Allows arterial closure at 'normal' arterial pressure → may reduce risk of post-op haematoma Disadvantages: • Risks associated with siting block • Patient stress/pain → increased risk of myocardial ischaemia • Restricted access to airway intra-operatively • Requires cooperative patient who is able to lie flat and still • Risk of conversion to general anaesthesia intra-operatively • Risk of local anaesthetic toxicity	Any 4 Any 4	*Whilst using general anaesthesia for CEA provides the surgeon with a still, cooperative patient, there are many disadvantages. The lack of direct intra-operative neurological monitoring means that surgeons are more likely to use shunts to prevent cerebral ischaemia during cross-clamping. Patients may be more haemodynamically unstable, with a hypertensive response at laryngoscopy and extubation, and hypotension intra-operatively.*

(cont.)

Q	Marking guidance	Mark	Comments
d	• Local anaesthetic infiltration alone	Any 2	
	• Deep cervical plexus block		*Usually performed in combination with a superficial cervical plexus block.*
	• Cervical epidural		*Rarely performed for CEA in the UK because of the risk of hypotension and serious complications.*
e	<u>Preparation:</u> • AAGBI-recommended standard monitoring • Awake arterial line in contralateral side • Intravenous access in contralateral side • Resuscitation equipment available • Trained assistant • Stop before you block <u>Block-specific:</u> • Superficial injection along posterior border of sternocleidomastoid • 10–15 mL of local anaesthetic, e.g. levobupivacaine 0.5% • Local anaesthetic is commonly injected in submandibular area	Any 5	Maximum of 3 marks for the block preparation. *As this is an area often 'missed' by this block.*
f	Diagnosis: cerebral hyperperfusion syndrome (CHS) Pathophysiology: ipsilateral loss of cerebral autoregulation leading to increased ipsilateral cerebral blood flow Management: aggressive blood pressure control	1 1 1	*CHS occurs in 1–3% of CEA patients. Risk factors include > 90% stenosis, intra-operative ischaemia or emboli. Seizures and cerebral oedema may result.*

Suggested reading

M. Lieb, U. Shah, G. L. Hines. Cerebral hyperperfusion syndrome after carotid intervention: a review. *Cardiol Rev* 2012; **20**(2): 84–9.

N. Ladak, J. Thompson. General or local anaesthesia for carotid endarterectomy? *Cont Edu Anaesth Crit Care Pain* 2012; **12**(2): 92–6.

S. J. Howell. Carotid endarterectomy. *Br J Anaesth* 2007; **99**(1): 119–31.

Question 12 Cardiopulmonary Exercise Testing

Q	Marking guidance	Mark	Comments
a	Resting = 1 MET Walking 2.5 mph = 2.9 METs (accept 3 METs) Climbing two flights stairs = 4 METs Jogging = 8 METs (accept 7–8 METs)	4	*A functional capacity of < 4 METs represents poor physiological fitness and is associated with a higher risk of perioperative complications.*
b	• Questionnaire-based, e.g. Duke Activity Status Index • Incremental shuttle walk • Six-min walk test • Step test	Any 3	*A 12-question self-assessment with each physical task weighted according to its MET. Patients walk continuously between two cones set 9 m apart with a progressively decreasing time permitted to reach the next cone. Distance walked in 6 min on the flat. Patients step up and down on a 20 cm step for 3 min.*
c	• Acute myocardial infarction • Unstable angina • Uncontrolled/symptomatic arrhythmia • Syncope • Active endocarditis • Acute myocarditis/pericarditis • Symptomatic severe aortic stenosis • Uncontrolled heart failure • Suspected dissecting or leaking aortic aneurysm • Uncontrolled asthma • Arterial desaturation at rest on room air <85%	Any 4	*Relative contraindications to CPET include:* • *Untreated left main stem disease* • *Asymptomatic severe aortic stenosis* • *Severe hypertension at rest* • *Hypertrophic cardiomyopathy* • *Pulmonary hypertension* • *Acute deep vein thrombosis* • *Abdominal aortic aneurysm > 8.0 cm*

(cont.)

Q	Marking guidance	Mark	Comments
d	• Increased heart rate • Increase in systolic blood pressure/decrease in diastolic blood pressure • Increase in minute ventilation • Increase in oxygen pulse Not acceptable: ECG changes (which are not recorded on the nine-panel plot) or metabolic gas exchange parameters	Any 3	*Oxygen pulse (VO_2/HR) is a surrogate for stroke volume which initially increases with exercise before reaching a plateau.*
e	• Peak oxygen consumption (VO_{2peak}) • Anaerobic threshold (AT) • Ventilatory efficiency for carbon dioxide	Any 2	*VO_{2peak} <15 $mLO_2/kg^{-1}/min$ and AT <11 $mLO_2/kg^{-1}/min$ are associated with poor post-operative outcomes.*
f	• Restoration of ATP and phosphocreatine stores • Restoration of myoglobin O_2 stores • Restoration of muscle and liver glycogen • Dissipation of heat • Restoration of intracellular electrolytes to normal concentrations • Repair/hypertrophy of muscle fibres	Any 4	*The excess post-exercise oxygen consumption (also known as oxygen debt) is the oxygen used in the processes that restore the body to its resting state and adapt it to the exercise just performed.*

Suggested reading

D. J. Chambers, N. Wisely. Cardiopulmonary exercise testing – a beginner's guide to the nine-panel plot. *BJA Educ, in press.*

D. Z. H. Levett, S. Jack, M. Swart, et al. Perioperative cardiopulmonary exercise testing (CPET): consensus clinical guidelines on indications, organisation, conduct, and physiological interpretation. *Br J Anaesth* 2018; **120**(3): 484–500.

N. Agnew. Preoperative cardiopulmonary exercise testing. *Cont Edu Anaesth Crit Care Pain* 2010; **10**(2): 33–7.

Paper 7 Answers

Question 1 Myasthenia Gravis

Q	Marking guidance	Mark	Comments
a	Symptoms: • Diplopia • Dysphagia • Dysarthria/nasal speech • Inability to smile/close mouth/ impaired facial expression • Difficulty chewing • Limb weakness • Dyspnoea	Any 4	*Due to weakness of extraocular muscles.* *Due to weakness of palatal/ pharyngeal muscles.* *Weakness of muscles of mastication.*
	Signs: • Fatigable weakness • Ptosis • External ophthalmoplegia/ strabismus (squint)	Any 2	*Weakness of levator palpebrae superioris.* *Weakness of extraocular muscles.*
b	Thymectomy (excision of thymoma)	1	
c	Nicotinic acetylcholine receptor Muscle-specific kinase (MuSK)	2	*Both of these are located at the neuromuscular junction.*
d	Immunoglobin-G (IgG)	1	*NB it must be IgG because autoantibodies can cross the placenta, resulting in congenital myasthenia gravis.*
e	• Autoimmune thyroiditis • Grave's disease • Rheumatoid arthritis • Type 1 diabetes mellitus • Scleroderma • Vitiligo • Polymyositis/dermatomyositis • Systemic lupus erythematosus • Pernicious anaemia	Any 3	*NB all these diseases are autoimmune in nature.*

(cont.)

Q	Marking guidance	Mark	Comments
f	Anticholinesterases	1	*E.g. pyridostigmine.*
	Immunosuppression	1	*E.g. prednisolone, azathioprine, cyclosporine.*
	Intravenous immunoglobulin or plasma exchange	1	
g	• Deep inhalational anaesthesia alone	Any 2	
	• Reduced dose of non-depolarising muscle relaxant		*~30% of normal dose of atracurium, vecuronium or rocuronium*
	• Increased dose of suxamethonium		
	• Remifentanil infusion/total intravenous anaesthesia		
h	• Inability to support head	Any 2	*Chin falls onto chest*
	• Absent gag reflex: risk of aspiration of oral secretions		
	• Poor or absent cough		*Accumulation of secretions*
	• Respiratory distress/use of accessory muscles/paradoxical abdominal breathing/ventilatory failure		

Suggested reading

M. Thavasothy, N. Hirsch. Myasthenia gravis. *BJA CEPD Reviews* 2002; **2**(3): 88–90.

Question 2   One-Lung Ventilation

Q	Marking guidance	Mark	Comments
a	White: Right Yes <u>Robertshaw:</u> Both No <u>Carlens:</u> Left Yes One mark for each correct paired answer	1 1 1	*The choice of double-lumen endotracheal tube (DLETT) size is based on patient height, gender and size of main stem bronchi. There is considerable variation in bronchial dimensions – in general, smaller tube sizes are best for females since the diameter of their cricoid cartilage is smaller than that of males.*
b	• Controlling distribution of ventilation, e.g. tracheobronchial tree injury/bronchopleural fistula • Avoiding cross-contamination of contralateral lung, e.g. endobronchial haemorrhage/abscess with empyema/bronchiectasis/lavage	1 1	Need both the indication and a correct example for a mark. *Surgical access is technically only a relative indication for one-lung ventilation!*
c	>1.5 L	1	*For pneumonectomy, an FEV_1 > 2 L is usually required*
d	>40% (accept 40%–50%)	1	*$\dot{V}/\dot{Q}$ scanning improves the accuracy of predicted post-operative ventilatory parameters as the pre-operative function of each lung may be taken into account.*
e	Maximal oxygen consumption (accept $\dot{V}O_{2\ max}$ or $\dot{V}O_{2\ peak}$) 15 mL/kg/min	1 1	*Recent literature suggests that patients with a pre-operative $\dot{V}O_{2\ max}$ >20 mL/kg/min are not at increased risk of complications or death; those with a $\dot{V}O_{2\ max}$ <10 mL/kg/min have a very high risk of post-operative complications.*

(cont.)

Q	Marking guidance	Mark	Comments
f	<u>Factors that increase pulmonary artery pressure:</u> • Atelectasis in the ventilated lung • Application of positive end-expiratory pressure (PEEP) in ventilated lung • Presence of intrinsic PEEP in the ventilated lung (e.g. asthma) • Diversion of blood to the non-ventilated lung (e.g. use of vasopressors) <u>Others:</u> • Failure of lung collapse • Use of vasodilators (e.g. inhalational anaesthesia, nitrates, calcium channel antagonists) • Turning to supine position	Any 3	Maximum of 2 marks from factors that increase pulmonary artery pressure.
g	• Administer 100% oxygen • Administer oxygen to the non-ventilated lung • Administer continuous positive airway pressure (CPAP) to the non-ventilated lung • Apply PEEP to the dependent lung • Ensure adequate haemoglobin/cardiac output • Revert to two lung ventilation • Nitric oxide • Consider high frequency jet ventilation	Any 6	*Clamping the non-dependent pulmonary artery is not an option here, as Mani is undergoing a lobectomy – not a pneumonectomy.*
h	<u>Advantage:</u> • May recruit collapsed alveoli <u>Disadvantage:</u> • May exacerbate shunt by impeding pulmonary blood flow to dependent lung • May reduce venous return with reduction in cardiac output	1 Any 1	

Suggested reading

A. Ng, J. Swanevelder. Hypoxaemia during one-lung anaesthesia. *Cont Edu Anaesth Crit Care Pain* 2010; **10**(4): 117–22.

B. Rippin, S. Kritzinger. One lung ventilation. World Federation of Societies of Anaesthesiologists' Anaesthesia Tutorial of the Week 145, 2009. www.aagbi.org/sites/default/files/145-One-lung-ventilation1.pdf. (Accessed 4 September 2018).

G. Gould, A. Pearce. Assessment of suitability for lung resection. *Cont Edu Anaesth Crit Care Pain* 2006; **6**(3): 97–100.

Question 3 Pulmonary Hypertension

Q	Marking guidance	Mark	Comments
a	Elevated mean pulmonary arterial pressure greater than or equal to 25 mmHg at rest	1	*PH is the most common cause of right ventricular failure.*
b	• Group 2: due to left heart disease • Group 3: due to lung disease or chronic hypoxia • Group 4: caused by pulmonary thromboemboli/other pulmonary artery obstructions • Group 5: due to haematological disorders, systemic disease and metabolic disorders	4	*Group 1 contains many subgroups, including familial, drug induced and those associated with medical conditions. Group 2 includes LV systolic or diastolic dysfunction, valvular heart disease and congenital heart defects. Group 3 includes chronic obstructive pulmonary disease, obstructive sleep apnoea and high-altitude exposure. Group 4 includes other pulmonary artery obstructions e.g. arteritis, stenosis, angiosarcoma. Group 5 includes haematological disorders (e.g. haemolysis), systemic disorders (e.g. sarcoidosis) and metabolic disorders (e.g. Gaucher's disease).*
c	• Raised jugular venous pressure • Peripheral oedema • Loud P2 • Right ventricular heave • Hepatomegaly • Irregular heart rate • Pansystolic murmur (tricuspid area)	Any 4	*The most common symptoms of PH are exertional shortness of breath, peripheral oedema and pre-syncope.*

(cont.)

Q	Marking guidance	Mark	Comments
d	• Right axis deviation • Dominant R wave in V1 • Dominant S wave in V6 • QRS < 120 ms • P pulmonale • Right ventricular strain pattern – ST depression or T-wave inversion in right precordial or inferior leads • Right bundle branch block	Any 3	*Other investigations: chest X-ray may show cardiomegaly and enlarged pulmonary arteries. Transthoracic echocardiogram: systolic pulmonary artery pressure > 36 mmHg is suggestive of PH.*
e	Tadalafil = phosphodiesterase V inhibitor → Increases c-GMP levels → NO is a potent vasodilator which acts via c-GMP	1 1 1	*Another phosphodiesterase V inhibitor is sildenafil. Both drugs are contra-indicated with systemic nitrates due to the risk of significant systemic hypotension.*
f	Treat underlying cause: E.g. antibiotics Optimise right ventricular (RV) preload: • Diuretics • Fluid therapy Reduce RV afterload: • Use of a prostanoid, sildenafil, inhaled nitric oxide • Avoid hypoxia/hypercapnoea, which exacerbate hypoxic pulmonary vasoconstriction Improve cardiac function: • Inotropes to improve RV contractility: dobutamine, dopamine, milrinone and enoximone • Consider venous–arterial ECMO	Any 5	 *In this context, optimising preload may mean diuretic therapy. Excess volume loading can reduce RV contractility leading to posterior bowing of the interventricular septum, which reduces left ventricular filling.* *Dobutamine is most commonly used, but may be limited by tachycardia and hypotension.*

(cont.)

Q	Marking guidance	Mark	Comments
	<u>Maintain perfusion pressure:</u> • Vasopressor to maintain systemic vascular resistance 1 mark for each principle, or an answer which exemplifies the principle		

Suggested reading

R. Condliffe, D. G. Kiely. Critical care management of pulmonary hypertension. *BJA Educ* 2017; **17**(7): 228–34.

Question 4   Post-tonsillectomy Haemorrhage

Q	Marking guidance	Mark	Comments
a	Primary: Occurring within 24 hours of surgery	1	The incidence of bleeding following tonsillectomy is 0.5%–2% depending upon the surgical technique.
	Secondary: Bleeding after 24 hours and up to 28 days post-surgery	1	The risk of haemorrhage increases with age, and is higher in males. A 'hot' surgical technique for both dissection and haemostasis (diathermy or radiofrequency coblation) has three times the risk of post-operative haemorrhage compared to traditional cold steel tonsillectomy.
b	• Ascending pharyngeal artery • Lesser palatine artery • Facial artery • Dorsal lingual artery • Ascending palatine artery • External carotid artery • Tonsillar artery	Any 2	Venous return is to the plexus around the tonsillar capsule, the lingual vein and the pharyngeal plexus. Post-tonsillectomy bleeding is usually venous in origin.

(cont.)

Q	Marking guidance	Mark	Comments
c	• Capillary refill time/peripheral pulses	Any 4	*Blood pressure is difficult to measure, especially in young children.*
			Hypotension is a late sign of hypovolaemia.
	• Respiratory rate		*Tachypnoea may be due to anxiety, but also occurs in response to the metabolic acidosis caused by poor tissue perfusion/severe anaemia.*
	• Core/peripheral temperature difference		*Core/skin temperature difference of more than 2°C is an important sign of shock.*
	• Urine output		*Poor urine output (<1 mL/kg/h in children, and <2 mL/kg/h in infants) indicates inadequate renal perfusion.*
	• Altered mental status		
	• Mottling/pallor/peripheral cyanosis		
d	• Aspiration risk (of regurgitated swallowed blood or post-operative oral intake)	Any 2	
	• Blood obscuring the laryngoscopic view		
	• Oedema from previous airway instrumentation and surgery		
e	Fluid: (accept any isotonic crystalloid)	Any 1	*Sam has no contraindications to receiving a 20 mL/kg bolus, i.e. no history of cardiac disease, renal disease or trauma. His haemoglobin is not sufficiently low to warrant transfusion at present.*
	• 0.9% Saline		
	• Hartmann's		
	• Plasmalyte 148		
	Volume:	1	
	400 mL (20 mL/kg)		

(cont.)

Q	Marking guidance	Mark	Comments
f	Technique: Inhalational induction in the head down, lateral position (must state head down or lateral positioning)	1	
	Advantages: • Drain blood from the airway by means of gravity • Allows for pre-oxygenation during induction	Any 1	
	Disadvantages: • Inhalational induction in an anxious child may be difficult • Deep inhalational anaesthesia risks cardiovascular instability in a potentially hypovolaemic child • Risk of laryngospasm/aspiration • Intubation in the lateral position is unfamiliar to most anaesthetists	Any 1	
	Technique: Rapid sequence induction	1	
	Advantages: • Reduced risk of aspiration • Use of muscle relaxants helps produce ideal conditions for intubation • Intravenous induction is less stressful for the child	Any 1	
	Disadvantages: • Difficult to adequately pre-oxygenate an anxious child who is bleeding • Facemask ventilation following muscle relaxant administration may inflate the stomach, increasing the risk of pulmonary aspiration • Potential for hypoxaemia if intubation is difficult (absence of spontaneous ventilation)	Any 1	

(cont.)

Q	Marking guidance	Mark	Comments
g	Accept any volume between 120 and 200 mL	1	*Two methods of determining volume:* *10 mL/kg = 200 mL* *Or* *Weight in kg × increment in Hb × 3* *The increment improvement here would be 2–3 g/dL to return Sam's Hb to a value > 8 g/dL. This equates to either 120 mL or 180 mL.*
h	24 hours	1	*Due to risk of rebleed.*

Suggested reading

D. Sethi, J. Smith. Anaesthesia for bleeding tonsil. World Federation of Societies of Anaesthesiologists' Anaesthesia Tutorial of the Week 51, 2007. www.aagbi.org/sites/defa ult/files/51-Anaesthesia-for-tonsillectomy .pdf. (Accessed 14 October 2018).

Question 5 Placental Abruption

Q	Marking guidance	Mark	Comments
a	• Anaemia • Infection • Maternal shock • Renal tubular necrosis • Coagulopathy • Post-partum haemorrhage (PPH) • Prolonged hospital stay • Psychological sequelae • Complications of transfusion • Sheehan's syndrome • Death	Any 5	*APH is defined as bleeding from or into the genital tract from 24 weeks until delivery of the baby.* *Causes of APH are placental abruption (one-third), placenta praevia (one-third) and 'other' (one-third).*
b	• Smoking • Cocaine use • Amphetamine use • Previous abruption • Previous uterine surgery/ previous caesarean section • Pre-eclampsia/hypertension • Extremes of maternal age: <25 years or >35 years • Multiparity • Thrombophilia • Trauma	Any 5	*Women who present with placental abruption alongside significant foetal compromise will be at risk of disseminated intravascular coagulation (DIC); bleeding may be concealed.*
c	• Systemic activation of coagulation leading to consumption of clotting factors • Leading to haemorrhage and/or thrombotic complications	1 1	*Widespread activation of coagulation leads to consumption of platelets and coagulation factors, increasing haemorrhage risk. Thrombotic complications result from intravascular fibrin formation.*

(cont.)

Q	Marking guidance	Mark	Comments
d	• Intrauterine death • Amniotic fluid embolus • Sepsis (obstetric source) • Pre-eclampsia • Retained products of conception • Induced abortion • Acute fatty liver	Any 5	*Non-obstetric causes include sepsis and severe infections, malignancy, vascular disorders and severe immunological reactions.*
e	• PT ratio <1.5 • Platelets >75 ×10^9/L (accept >50×10^9/L) • Fibrinogen >2 g/L • Ionised calcium >1 mmol/L • Temperature >36°C • Hb >80 g/L (accept >70 g/L)	1 mark for 2 correct answers	

Suggested reading

F. Plaat, A. Shonfeld. Major obstetric haemorrhage. *BJA Educ* 2015; **15**(4): 190–3.
Royal College of Obstetricians and Gynaecologists. Antepartum Haemorrhage: RCOG Green-top Guideline No. 63, 2011. www.rcog.org.uk/en/guidelines-research-services/guidelines/gtg63. (Accessed 14 October 2018).

Question 6 Fascia Iliaca Block

Q	Marking guidance	Mark	Comments
a	Femoral Obturator Lateral cutaneous nerve of the thigh Sciatic	4	*A fascia iliaca block should anaesthetise all but the sciatic nerve.*
b	• Offer immediate analgesia on presentation • Regular assessment of pain • Ensure analgesia is sufficient to allow movements necessary for clinical examination • Offer regular paracetamol • Offer opioids if paracetamol insufficient • Non-steroidal anti-inflammatory drugs are not recommended	Any 4	*Pain should be assessed on arrival at the Emergency Department, within 30 min of administering analgesia and hourly until settled on the ward.* *Adequate analgesia is indicated by the ability to tolerate passive external rotation of the leg.*
c	• Analgesia for hip surgery • Analgesia for above knee amputation • Analgesia for plaster administration in children with femoral fracture • Analgesia for knee surgery • Analgesia for lower leg tourniquet pain	Any 3	*In combination with a sciatic nerve block, a fascia iliaca block provides analgesia for knee and lower leg surgery.*
d	• 'WHO' sign in (confirm patient identity, consent and marking of surgical site) • Subsequent check immediately before needle insertion of: • Surgical site marking AND side of block (side of block can be confirmed with patient or consent form) • Two-person check	1 1 1 1	*Wrong site nerve blocks are associated with* • *delays in performing the surgical procedure* • *turning the patient* • *lower limb blocks* • *trainee operators* • *distraction*

(cont.)

Q	Marking guidance	Mark	Comments
e	• Draw line between anterior superior iliac spine and pubic tubercle • Insertion point 1 cm caudal to the junction of lateral and middle thirds of this line • Palpate femoral artery to ensure it is medial and away from site of insertion • Insert needle at 60° cranial angle • 'Two-pop' technique using blunt needle	Any 4	*The two 'pops' refer to passing through the fascia lata and the fascia iliaca. Traversing these fascial layers is more pronounced when using a blunt needle. The ultrasound-guided approach has been found to be superior to the landmark-guided approach.*
f	Previous femoral bypass surgery	1	

Suggested reading

C. Range, C. Egeler. Fascia iliaca compartment block. World Federation of Societies of Anaesthesiologists' Anaesthesia Tutorial of the Week 193. 2010. www.aagbi.org/sites/def ault/files/193-Fascia-Iliaca-compartment-blo ck.pdf. (Accessed 14 October 2018).

National Institute for Health and Care Excellence. Pathway – hip fracture overview. 2018. http://pathways .nice.org.uk/pathways/hip-fracture. (Accessed 14 October 2018).

Question 7   Paracetamol Overdose

Q	Marking guidance	Mark	Comments
a	• Paracetamol is metabolised by the liver	1	*Toxicity is dose dependent:*
	• A minor metabolite is *N*-acetyl-p-benzoquinoneimine (NAPQI) which is toxic/reactive	1	*• <150 mg/kg taken over a period of > 1 hour is unlikely to cause toxicity*
			• >12 g has the potential to be fatal
	• Glutathione normally conjugates NAPQI	1	*NAPQI binds to cellular proteins causing hepatocyte damage.*
	• In overdose, glutathione stores are depleted	1	*N-acetyl cysteine (NAC) is a precursor of glutathione and replenishes stores.*
b	• Nausea/vomiting • Abdominal pain • Coma	Any 2	*Aside from nausea and vomiting, symptoms within the first 24 hours are rare. Coma may occur with plasma concentration > 800 mg/L.*
c	• Presentation within 1 hour of overdose	1	*The benefits of gastric decontamination are unclear, but activated charcoal remains in the Toxbase recommendations following paracetamol overdose.*
	• Dose taken > 150 mg/kg	1	
d	• Malnourished/cachexia • Eating disorders • Alcoholism • Hepatic enzyme induction • Chronic liver disease • Chronic kidney disease	Any 4	

(cont.)

Q	Marking guidance	Mark	Comments
e	Diagnosis: anaphylactoid reaction Management: • Stop the infusion • Chlorphenamine • Salbutamol nebuliser • Restart infusion at a slower rate	1 Any 3	*Anaphylactoid reactions to intravenous NAC are common, occurring in up to 30% of patients, and are usually associated with the first exposure to NAC and rapid infusion rates. Previous anaphylactoid reactions are not a contraindication to treatment with NAC.*
f	Prediction model: King's College criteria Criteria: • pH < 7.3 • INR > 6 (accept PT > 100 s) • Creatinine > 300 µmol/L • Encephalopathy grade 3 or 4	1 Any 3	*King's College criteria are the most widely used in the UK. Liver transplantation is considered if the pH is less than 7.3, or all three of the remaining criteria are present within a 24-hour period.*

Suggested reading

P. Maclure, B. Salman. Management of acute liver failure in critical care. World Federation of Societies of Anaesthesiologists' Anaesthesia Tutorial of the Week 251. 2012. www.aagbi.org/sites/default/files/251%20Acute%20Liver%20Failure%20in%20Critical%20Care[2].pdf. (Accessed 31 October 2018).

Question 8 Carcinoid Syndrome

Q	Marking guidance	Mark	Comments
a	• Flushing • Lacrimation • Rhinorrhoea	Any 2	*Carcinoid syndrome is typically intermittent. It is associated with exercise, the ingestion of alcohol or high tyramine content foods such as blue cheeses and chocolate.*
b	Enterochromaffin cells (accept Kulchitsky cells)	1	*Carcinoid tumours arise from the different embryonic divisions of the gut. Foregut tumours arise in the lungs, bronchi or stomach; midgut tumours occur in the small intestine, appendix and proximal colon, and hindgut carcinoid tumours arise in the distal colon or rectum.*
c	• Serotonin • Corticotrophin • Histamine • Dopamine • Substance P • Neurotensin • Prostaglandins • Kallikrein	Any 3	
d	Tricuspid valve Pulmonary valve	1 1	*Carcinoid heart disease classically affects the right side of the heart with fibrous thickening of the endocardium causing retraction and fixation of the tricuspid valve leaflets. Fibrosis is related to the duration of exposure to high concentrations of 5-hydroxytryptamine.*

(cont.)

Q	Marking guidance	Mark	Comments
e	Somatostatin	1	*Octreotide has widespread side effects: QT prolongation, bradycardia, conduction defects and vomiting.*
f	Advantage: Avoidance of stressors such as pain reduces risk of carcinoid crisis Disadvantage: Exaggerated response to vasopressors used to counteract neuraxial blockade-induced hypotension	1 1	*The balance of risks would seem to favour the use of epidurals with vasopressors cautiously titrated to response.*
g	• Arterial line • Central line • Cardiac output monitoring • Bispectral index/depth of anaesthesia	Any 3	
h	• Hypertension (accept 'fluctuating blood pressure'; only 1 mark to be awarded for blood pressure related response) • Bronchospasm (accept change in capnography trace/increase in ventilatory pressures) • Tachycardia • Sweating Octreotide dose: 20–50 µg	Any 3 1	*The most common causes of carcinoid crises are anaesthetic, radiological or surgical interventions. Carcinoid crisis is potentially fatal.*
i	Safe: • Phenylephrine • Vasopressin Extreme caution: Adrenergic agents	Any 1 1	*The response to vasopressors is unpredictable and drugs such as norepinephrine and epinephrine can be hazardous.* *Norepinephrine has been shown to activate kallikrein in the tumour and can lead*

Q	Marking guidance	Mark	Comments
			to the synthesis and release of bradykinin, resulting paradoxically in vasodilatation and worsening hypotension. Exaggerated hypertensive responses to epinephrine and norepinephrine may also be seen.

Suggested reading

B. Powell, A. Mukhtar, G H Mills. Carcinoid: the disease and its implications for anaesthesia. *Cont Edu Anaesth Crit Care Pain* 2011; 11(1): 9–13.

Question 9 Diabetes Day Case

Q	Marking guidance	Mark	Comments
a	69 mmol/mol (accept 70 mmol/mol or 8.5%)	1	*The AAGBI guidelines recommend delaying elective surgery if HbA1c is ≥ 69 mmol/mol, as poor diabetic control is associated with increased perioperative complications.*
b	ECG Urea and electrolytes	1 1	*A random blood glucose is NOT required.* *An HbA1c taken within the last 3 months is required.*
c	Metformin: Mechanism: • Delays gut glucose uptake • Increases peripheral insulin sensitivity • Inhibits gluconeogenesis Dose day of surgery: normal Gliclazide: Mechanism: • Displaces insulin from β-cells • Reduces peripheral insulin resistance Dose day of surgery: omit Dapagliflozin: Mechanism: • Sodium–glucose co-transporter type 2 (SGLT2) inhibitor • Increases urinary glucose excretion Dose day of surgery: halve (accept omit)	Any 1 1 Any 1 1 Any 1 1	*Dose alterations may be needed for the following oral diabetic medication classes:* • *Meglitinides (e.g. repaglinide, nateglinide)* • *Sulphonylureas (e.g. glibenclamide, gliclazide, glipizide)* • *SGLT-2 inhibitors (e.g. dapagliflozin, canagliflozin)* • *Acarbose* *On rare occasions, SGLT2 inhibitors have been associated with ketoacidosis in fasting patients, therefore the 2015 AAGBI guidelines recommend halving the dose on the day of surgery. Subsequently, omission of SGLT2 has been recommended.*

Q	Marking guidance	Mark	Comments
d	Target: 6–10 mmol/L (accept 6–12 mmol/L)	1	*A blood glucose measurement should be taken prior to induction of anaesthesia.*
	Frequency: hourly	1	
e	Blood glucose 17 mmol/L:		*0.1 IU/kg to a maximum of 6 IU should be used to manage hyperglycaemia in patients with type 2 diabetes who do not normally take insulin.*
	Drug: Insulin	1	
	Dose: 0.1 IU/kg (accept 6 IU)	1	
	Blood glucose 2.6 mmol/L:		
	Drug: IV glucose/dextrose	1	
	Dose: 100 mL of 20% glucose (accept 20 g)	1	
f	Advantages:	Any 2	
	• Reduced incidence of post-operative nausea and vomiting		
	• Earlier return to oral medication		
	• Opioid sparing		*Resulting in reduced opioid side effects.*
	• May reduce catabolic hormone release		
	• Reduced risk of pulmonary aspiration		*Diabetic autonomic neuropathy may put diabetic patients at risk of aspiration during general anaesthesia.*
	Disadvantages:	Any 2	
	• Increased risk of epidural/spinal abscess		*Due to diabetes-related immunosuppression.*
	• Increased risk of haemodynamic instability		*Due to autonomic neuropathy.*
	• Increased risk of peripheral neuropathy		*Due to diabetic neuropathy.*

(cont.)

Q	Marking guidance	Mark	Comments
g	4 hours	1	*Dexamethasone should be avoided in patients with diabetes unless the risk of post-operative nausea and vomiting outweighs the risk of hyperglycaemia.*

Suggested reading

D. J. Stubbs, N. Levy, K. Dhatariya. Diabetes medication pharmacology. *BJA Educ* 2017; **17**(6): 198–207.

P. Barker, P. E. Creasey, K. Dhatariya, et al. Perioperative management of the surgical patient with diabetes. *Anaesthesia* 2015; **70**(12): 1427–40.

Question 10   Traumatic Pelvic and Brain Injury

Q	Marking guidance	Mark	Comments
a	Best eye response	1	
	Best verbal response	1	
	Best motor response	1	
b	Haemorrhage	1	*A heart rate of 125 beats/ min and systolic blood pressure of 92 mmHg suggest class III shock.*
c	• Airway protection • Reduced conscious level/GCS < 8 • To prevent secondary brain injury • To protect the cervical spine • To allow for safe radiological imaging	Any 3	*I.e. to prevent hypercapnoea and hypoxaemia* *~10% incidence of cervical spinal fractures in patients with severe traumatic brain injury.*
d	• Intravenous access • Oxygen • Administer blood products • Diagnosis of head injury (CT head) • Diagnosis of haemorrhage (CT trauma series: cervical spine, thorax, abdomen, pelvis) • General surgical review • Pelvic binder/X-rays • Focussed Assessment with Sonography for Trauma (FAST) scan • Patient warming • Intravenous tranexamic acid	Any 4	*Wide-bore, multiple.* *Group O negative blood, send patient blood samples for cross-matched/group-specific blood.* *CRASH-2 trial: early tranexamic acid reduced mortality due to bleeding in trauma.*

(cont.)

Q	Marking guidance	Mark	Comments
e	• Mastoid ecchymosis (Battle's sign) • Periorbital ecchymosis (raccoon eyes) • Cerebrospinal fluid rhinorrhoea • Cerebrospinal fluid otorrhoea • Haematotympanum • VII cranial nerve palsy • VIII cranial nerve palsy	Any 4	
f	• Haematuria • Blood at the urethral meatus • Extravasated urine in the scrotum/subcutaneous tissue of penis • High-riding prostate	Any 2	
g	• Interventional radiology/embolisation of bleeding vessel • Initiate major haemorrhage alert/further blood products/intravenous tranexamic acid • Pelvic binder • External fixation of pelvis • Pelvic packing • Point-of-care coagulation testing	Any 3	*Major haemorrhage in the pelvis can be difficult to control due to bleeding directly into a free space potentially capable of accommodating a patient's entire blood volume without gaining sufficient pressure for a tamponade effect.*

Suggested reading

M. A. Akuji, E. E. Chapman, P. A. D. Clements. Anaesthesia for the management of traumatic pelvic fractures. *BJA Educ* 2018; **18**(7): 204–10.

Question 11 Post-thyroidectomy Haematoma

Q	Marking guidance	Mark	Comments
a	• Duration of goitre • Able to lie flat • Positional dyspnoea/stridor • Change in voice • Is it possible to feel below the thyroid gland? • Tracheal deviation • Signs of superior vena cava obstruction	Any 6	*A large, long-standing goitre is a risk factor for post-operative tracheomalacia.* *Retrosternal thyroid.* *Pemberton's sign: asking the patient to raise his or her arms – obstruction results in the patient's face becoming blue and engorged.*
b	• Thyroid function tests • Full blood count • Chest X-ray/CT neck and thorax • Nasendoscopy • Spirometry • ECG	Any 4	*It is important to ensure the patient is biochemically euthyroid prior to surgery to avoid complications such as intra-operative thyroid storm.* *A pre-operative haemoglobin concentration is indicated due to the risk of intra-operative bleeding.* *To exclude tracheal deviation and retrosternal extension of the thyroid gland.* *Routinely performed by ENT surgeons to document pre-operative vocal cord function.* *Flow-volume loops may demonstrate fixed upper airway obstruction.*

(cont.)

Q	Marking guidance	Mark	Comments
c	• Laryngeal oedema • Post-extubation laryngospasm • Tracheomalacia • Unilateral recurrent laryngeal nerve palsy Not acceptable: acute hypocalcaemia, which may cause laryngospasm but ionised calcium does not fall to that extent within this timescale	4	*Bilateral recurrent laryngeal nerve palsy will be apparent immediately after extubation, as there is complete adduction of both vocal cords and stridor.*
d	• Administer oxygen • Removal of surgical clips/sutures to release haematoma • Sit patient up • Return to theatre • ENT surgeon on standby for awake tracheostomy • Anticipate difficult airway/prepare difficult airway equipment/smaller endotracheal tube than previous intubation	Any 4	*Removal of surgical clips allows decompression of the haematoma and often relieves stridor, permitting a less fraught anaesthetic induction. However, a neck haematoma often impairs laryngeal venous drainage, resulting in laryngeal oedema. The airway may therefore still be challenging.*
e	Valsalva manoeuvre: • Switch to manual ventilation • Close APL valve • Gently squeeze reservoir bag until airway pressure is 20–30 cmH$_2$0 • Hold for 10 seconds Purpose: Increased intrathoracic pressure increases venous pressure. Venous or capillary bleeding will become brisker and hence more obvious to the surgeon	1 1	*This manoeuvre is known as a 'passive Valsalva manoeuvre'. A true Valsalva manoeuvre, which involves forced expiration against a closed glottis, cannot be replicated under general anaesthesia.*

Suggested reading

S. Malhotra, V. Sodhi. Anaesthesia for thyroid and parathyroid surgery. *Cont Edu Anaesth Crit Care Pain* 2007; 7(2): 55–8.

L. Adams, S. Davies. Anaesthesia for thyroid surgery. World Federation of Societies of Anaesthesiologists' Anaesthesia Tutorial of the Week 162, 2009. www .aagbi.org/sites/default/files/162-Anaesthesia-for-thyroid-surgery.pdf. (Accessed 18 August 2018).

Question 12 Vagus Nerve

Q	Marking guidance	Mark	Comments
a	Dorsal nucleus of the vagus	Any 2	*Sends parasympathetic output to the viscera, especially the intestine.*
	Nucleus ambiguus		*Motor fibres to pharynx, soft palate and larynx, and parasympathetic output to the heart.*
	Nucleus tractus solitarius		*Receives sensory information from viscera.*
b	• Anterior: right lobe of thyroid gland • Posterior: longus cervicis or anterior scalene muscle • Medial: common carotid artery • Lateral: internal jugular vein	Any 3	NB this question asks about the **immediate** relations to the vagus nerve
c	• Anterior: superior vena cava or azygos vein • Posterior: right lung or oesophagus • Medial: trachea • Lateral: azygos vein or brachiocephalic vein	Any 3	NB this question asks about the **immediate** relations to the vagus nerve
d	• Small meningeal nerve • Auricular nerve • Pharyngeal nerve • Carotid body branches • Superior laryngeal nerve • Recurrent laryngeal nerve • Superior and inferior cardiac branches • Anterior and posterior bronchial branches • Anterior vagal trunk • Posterior vagal trunk	Any 6	*'Vagus' is from the Latin meaning 'wandering'. The vagus supplies a large number of viscera during its wandering course through the neck, thorax and abdomen.*

(cont.)

Q	Marking guidance	Mark	Comments
e	T10	1	*The vagus nerve traverses the diaphragm through the oesophageal hiatus.*
f	Treatment resistant epilepsy Treatment resistant depression	2	
g	Surgical diathermy: • Avoid, or use bipolar diathermy • If monopolar diathermy is absolutely necessary, place earth plate as far away as possible from stimulator box/leads Defibrillation: • Place electrode pads perpendicular to, and as far away as possible from the device Nerve stimulator: • Nerve localisation using a peripheral nerve stimulator may interfere with the vagal nerve stimulator	Any 2	*Just like an implanted cardiac device, vagal nerve stimulators have implications for surgery and for magnetic resonance imaging.* *Most anaesthetists now use ultrasound-guided techniques for nerve blocks.*

Suggested reading

P.-S. Whitney, J. Sturgess. Anaesthetic considerations for patients with neurosurgical implants. *BJA Educ* 2016; **16**(7): 230–5.

Paper 8 Answers

Question 1 Scoliosis

Q	Marking guidance	Mark	Comments
a	Lateral curvature and rotation (accept abnormal curvature) of thoracolumbar vertebrae (accept spinal column)	1 1	*Scoliosis is defined as the lateral curvature and rotation of the thoracolumbar vertebrae, leading to rib cage deformity.*
b	• Neuromuscular disorders: cerebral palsy, myopathies, poliomyelitis, syringomyelia, Friedrich's ataxia • Congenital: vertebral anomalies, rib anomalies, spinal dysraphism • Traumatic: fractures, radiation, surgery • Syndromes: Marfan's, rheumatoid, osteogenesis imperfecta, mucopolysaccharidoses, neurofibromatosis • Malignancy • Infection: tuberculosis, osteomyelitis	Any 4 Max 2 from any category	*Surgery is performed to prevent progression of the disease.* *Depending on aetiology, further investigations may be required prior to surgery.*
c	Cobb angle 40° (accept 40°–50°)	1 1	*Cobb angle > 10° is abnormal.*
d	Respiratory: • CXR • Lung function tests Cardiac: • ECG • Echocardiogram	 1 1 1 1	*Cobb angle > 65° will impede respiratory function. Cobb angle > 100° can lead to respiratory failure, pulmonary hypertension and right heart failure.*

Q	Marking guidance	Mark	Comments
e	• Somatosensory evoked potentials (SSEPs) and motor evoked potentials (MEPs) • SSEPs stimulate peripheral nerve and detect response with epidural/scalp electrode • SSEPs evaluate the integrity of ascending sensory tracts • MEPs stimulate motor cortex and detect response with epidural electrodes/compound motor action potentials (CMAPs) • MEPs are designed to evaluate the integrity of descending motor tracts • Nerve injury: indicated by decrease in amplitude/latency of SSEPs or loss of CMAPs in MEPs	Any 4	*An increase in SSEP latency of > 10% and decrease in amplitude of > 50% is considered significant. MEPs: a transient loss of CMAPs may not indicate nerve injury, but complete loss of CMAPs should be taken seriously.*
f	• Propofol • Volatile agents • Nitrous oxide • Muscle relaxants Only one mark given per drug class	4	*SSEPs are affected by propofol, volatile agents and nitrous oxide. MEPs are affected by propofol, volatile agents, nitrous oxide and muscle relaxants. A decrease in blood pressure and temperature may also affect signals.*

Suggested reading

M. A. Entwistle, D. Patel. Scoliosis surgery in children. *Cont Edu Anaesth Crit Care Pain* 2006; **6**(1): 13–6.

J. M. Kynes, F. M. Evans. Surgical correction of scoliosis: anaesthetic considerations. World Federation of Societies of Anaesthesiologists' Anaesthesia Tutorial of the Week 318, 2015. www.aagbi.org/sites/default/files/318%20Sur gical%20Correction%20of%20Scoliosis.pdf. (Accessed 17 October 2018).

Question 2 Cardiac Bypass

Q	Marking guidance	Mark	Comments
a	i = aortic cross-clamp ii = venous reservoir iii = systemic blood pump iv = vent pump (accept 'vent') v = cardiotomy reservoir vi = gas exchanger (accept 'oxygenator') vii = cardioplegia solution (accept 'cardioplegia')	7	
b	Heparin 300–400 IU/kg Target ACT: >480 seconds	1 1	*ACT monitors the anticoagulant effect of unfractionated heparin.*
c	Potassium inactivates fast inward sodium channels, preventing the upstroke of the myocyte action potential	1	*This renders the myocardium unexcitable and in diastolic arrest. Cardioplegia can be administered by an anterograde approach (via the aortic root, provided aortic valve is competent), via a retrograde approach (via the coronary sinus), or both. It is usually delivered intermittently (every 15–30 min).*
d	• Oxygen carrying capacity • Hydrogen ion buffering • Free-radical scavenging • Improved microvascular flow • Reduced myocardial oedema • Delivery of other nutrients	Any 3	*Glutamate and aspartate are sometimes added to cardioplegia to promote oxidative metabolism in energy-depleted hearts.*
e	Advantages: • Reduced cerebral oxygen consumption/reduced cerebral ischaemia (accept 'cerebral protection')	Any 4	*More challenging operations may require deep hypothermia (15°–22°C) to allow periods of low blood flow or deep hypothermic circulatory*

Q	Marking guidance	Mark	Comments
	• Reduces myocardial oxygen consumption • Decreases rate of release of neurotransmitters associated with neuronal death • Reduced inflammatory response • Reduced blood–brain barrier permeability • Improved organ protection		*arrest (DHCA). Circulatory arrest is typically undertaken at 18°–20°C. Most patients tolerate 30 minutes of DHCA without significant neurological injury. Longer periods of DHCA are tolerated better by neonates and infants compared with adults.*
	Disadvantages: • Increased blood viscosity (accept 'increased embolic risk') • Increased infection risk • Impaired wound healing • Peripheral vasoconstriction • Impairs liberation of O_2 from haemoglobin • Increased bleeding risk/ impaired coagulation • Hyperglycaemia • Metabolic acidosis • Cardiac arrhythmias	Any 3	*At a biochemical level, changes in temperature alter reaction rates and metabolic processes by a factor known as the Q10 effect, which defines the amount of increase or decrease in these processes relative to a 10°C difference in temperature.*

Suggested reading

D. Machin, C. Allsager. Principles of cardiopulmonary bypass. *Cont Edu Anaesth Crit Care Pain* 2006; **6**(5): 176–81.

Question 3   Guillain–Barré Syndrome

Q	Marking guidance	Mark	Comments
a	Acute demyelinating polyneuropathy	1	*It is an autoimmune phenomenon, usually following a gastrointestinal or respiratory infection. This infection may be very minor.*
b	• Motor: progressive, usually ascending, motor weakness • Reflexes: areflexia • Cranial nerves: facial nerve palsy, bulbar weakness • Eyes: ophthalmoplegia, ptosis, diplopia • Sensory symptoms: pain, numbness, paraesthesia • Respiratory: respiratory muscle weakness → respiratory failure • Autonomic dysfunction: arrhythmias, labile blood pressure, urinary retention, paralytic ileus and hyperhidrosis	Any 5	*Several clinical pictures of GBS are described, including* *– Acute inflammatory demyelinating polyradiculopathy (most common)* *– Acute motor axonal neuropathy* *– Acute motor and sensory axonal neuropathy* *– Miller Fisher syndrome (affects eyes but not always accompanied by limb weakness)* *Usually ascending sensory loss. 'Glove and stocking' distribution also seen.* *GBS often has a variable presentation and should be suspected in any patient with unexplainable weakness or sensory deficit affecting the limbs.*

(cont.)

Q	Marking guidance	Mark	Comments
c	• Nausea • Fever • Headache • Transient rise in liver enzymes • Encephalopathy • Meningism • Malaise • Erythroderma • Hypercoagulability • Renal tubular necrosis • Anaphylaxis	Any 4	*Side effects (<5% of patients) are usually mild.*
d	Plasmapheresis/plasma exchange	1	*Plasmapheresis reduces the duration of ventilator dependence and hospital stay, and leads to earlier mobilisation if commenced within 2 weeks of the onset of illness.*
e	• Vital capacity < 15–20 mL/kg • Maximum inspiratory pressure < 30 cmH$_2$O • Maximum expiratory pressure < 40 cmH$_2$O • Bulbar involvement • Respiratory failure on arterial blood gas (rising P_aCO$_2$) • Significant autonomic instability	6	*Deterioration in respiratory function may be rapid: patients should have vital capacity measured three times daily.* *Impairs cough and ability to protect the airway.*
f	• *Campylobacter* spp. infection • Old age • Need for ventilatory support • Anti-GM1 antibody • Neurone specific enolase • S-100 proteins in the cerebrospinal fluid • Absent or reduced compound muscle action potential • Inexcitable nerves • Upper limb paralysis	Any 3	

Suggested reading

K. J. C. Richards, T. Cohen. Guillain–Barré
  syndrome. *Br J Anaesth CEPD
  Reviews* 2003; **3**(2): 46–9.

Question 4 Meningitis

Q	Marking guidance	Mark	Comments
a	• Headache • Neck stiffness • Nausea/vomiting • Photophobia • Drowsiness • Coma • Seizures	Any 4	
b	Weight: 'Old' formula: (age+4) × 2 = 12 kg 'New' formula: (age×2) + 8 = 12 kg Heart rate: 80–140 beats/min Systolic blood pressure: 85–100 mmHg Capillary refill < 2 seconds	1 1 1 1	
c	• ABCDE assessment • Early administration of broad-spectrum antibiotics, e.g. ceftriaxone • Oxygen • Fluid resuscitation • Dexamethasone • Prepare for intubation	Any 4	*In the pre-hospital setting, intravenous or intramuscular benzylpenicillin is indicated.*

(cont.)

Q	Marking guidance	Mark	Comments
d	<u>Investigation</u>: CT scan of brain	1	*CT imaging is carried out to exclude complications of bacterial meningitis that may make lumbar puncture risky, most commonly subdural collections in H. influenzae, meningitis, and obstructive hydrocephalus in M. tuberculosis meningitis.*
	<u>Results:</u> • Most commonly normal appearance • Subdural collection • Obstructive hydrocephalus • Leptomeningeal enhancement (accept meningeal enhancement) • Evidence of raised intracranial pressure e.g. effacement of ventricles	Any 2	
	<u>Investigation</u>: lumbar puncture	1	*In a child with neurological signs, lumbar puncture should only be performed after CT has excluded causes of raised intracranial pressure. Otherwise, lumbar puncture potentially risks precipitating cerebellar herniation.*
	<u>Results:</u> • Cloudy and turbid cerebrospinal fluid • Elevated opening pressure • Raised white cell count • Elevated protein • Low glucose • Culture: gram negative diplococci	Any 2	
e	• *Haemophilus influenzae* type B • *Streptococcus pneumoniae* • Group B *Streptococcus* • *Mycobacterium tuberculosis*	Any 2	*Asking about the child's immunisation history is important.*

Suggested reading

P. B. Baines, C. A. Hart. Severe meningococcal disease in childhood. *Br J Anaesth* 2003; **90**(1): 72–83.

Question 5   Puerperal Sepsis

Q	Marking guidance	Mark	Comments
a	• Obesity • Diabetes/impaired glucose tolerance • Immunosuppression • Anaemia • History of pelvic infection • Amniocentesis • Cervical cerclage • Prolonged rupture of membranes • Group A streptococcal infection in family members • Black or minority ethnic group	Any 5	*The management of maternal sepsis comprises a bundle of measures:* • *High-flow oxygen* • *Blood cultures* • *Broad-spectrum antibiotics* • *Fluid resuscitation* • *Serum lactate measurement* • *Catheterisation*
b	• Cardiovascular stability	1	*Septic, vasodilated patients may not tolerate a sympathetic block well.*
	• Infection risk	1	*Includes risk of epidural abscess and meningitis.*
	• Haematoma risk	1	*An associated coagulopathy will increase the risk of haematoma formation.*
c	• Urinary tract infection • Mastitis • Pneumonia • Skin/soft tissue • Gastroenteritis • Pharyngitis	Any 5	*Causes of genital tract sepsis include:* • *Chorioamnionitis* • *Endometritis* • *Septic abortion* • *Wound infection (vaginal tear, episiotomy, caesarean section)*
d	Pathogen: Group A *Streptococcus* Laboratory tests: • Throat swab • Blood cultures	1 1 1	*Other major pathogens: E. coli, influenza, S. aureus (methicillin-sensitive and resistant), S. pneumoniae, Clostridium septicum, Morganella morganii.*

(cont.)

Q	Marking guidance	Mark	Comments
e	• Early warning score system modified for obstetric use • Access to critical care support • Where possible, escalation should not lead to separation of mother and baby • Named consultant anaesthetist and obstetrician responsible for the woman's care 24 hours per day • Women requiring critical care in a non-obstetric facility should be reviewed daily by an obstetric team • Midwives providing a level of care beyond their routine scope of practice should be appropriately trained • NICE guidance on acute illness in adults should be implemented	Any 4	*The GPAS guidelines are intended to define the standards for the provision of anaesthetic care in all UK consultant-led maternity units. They discuss staffing, equipment and facilities, training and education and care for patients with special requirements. This includes care for the acutely ill obstetric patient as well as care for obese women and patients under the age of 18.*

Suggested reading

R. J. Elton, S. Chaudhari. Sepsis in obstetrics. *Cont Edu Anaesth Crit Care Pain* 2015; **15**(5): 259–64.

Royal College of Obstetricians and Gynaecologists. Bacterial Sepsis following Pregnancy: RCOG Green-top Guideline No. 64B. 2012. www.rcog.org.uk/en/guidelines-research-services/guidelines/gtg64b/. (Accessed 17 October 2018).

D. Bogod, F. Plaat, M. Mushambi, et al. Guidelines for the Provision of Anaesthesia Services for an Obstetric Population, 2018. In: *Guidelines for the Provision of Anaesthesia Services*. Royal College of Anaesthetists. www.rcoa.ac.uk/system/files/GPAS-2018–09-OBSTETRICS.pdf. (Accessed 17 October 2018).

Question 6 Brachial Plexus

Q	Marking guidance	Mark	Comments
a	C5, C6, C7, C8 and T1 (accept C5–T1)	1	
b	Approach → level Interscalene → roots Supraclavicular → trunks (accept proximal divisions) Infraclavicular → cords Axillary → terminal branches (accept branches)	1 2 1 2	*The interscalene block is most commonly used for shoulder and upper arm surgery. It is the only brachial plexus approach that reliably blocks the suprascapular nerve. It has limited use in lower arm surgery due to the C8/T1 ulnar component often being missed.*
c	• Horner's syndrome (accept stellate ganglion block) • Hoarseness (accept recurrent laryngeal nerve block) • Epidural/intrathecal spread of anaesthesia/total spinal anaesthesia • Intervertebral artery injection/seizures • Direct spinal cord damage from needle	Any 4	*Phrenic nerve palsy occurs in nearly 100% of interscalene blocks, and therefore has not been listed here as a complication – it is rather a well-recognised side effect.*
d	50 mm needle	1	*A short needle helps improve safety of the block as the brachial plexus is very superficial when performing an interscalene approach.*
e	• The trunks of the brachial plexus are located in the interscalene groove (accept between anterior and middle scalene muscles) • The ultrasound probe is usually placed at the level of C6 (accept C5–C7)	1 1	

(cont.)

Q	Marking guidance	Mark	Comments
f	• Accuracy of needle placement • Visualisation of degree of local anaesthetic spread • Compensation for anatomical variation/approach not landmark dependent • Rapid block onset • Reduced volume of local anaesthesia required • Reduced procedural pain/ improved patient satisfaction	Any 3	*There is level 1b evidence available to demonstrate that ultrasound guidance improves both the quality and the speed of block onset. Dynamic visualisation of the relevant anatomical structures and needle along with observation of local anaesthetic spread in real time are arguably the biggest advantages of ultrasound-guided regional anaesthesia.*
g	• Difficulty with patient positioning • Variable anatomy • Potential respiratory involvement may increase risk of respiratory embarrassment with phrenic nerve palsy • May have existing peripheral neurological deficit	Any 3	*Patients with rheumatoid arthritis merit special consideration as atlantoaxial instability is found in ~25% of sufferers. Therefore, regional anaesthesia as the sole technique is always worth considering to avoid laryngoscopy or other airway manoeuvres.*

Suggested reading

C. Beecroft, D. M. Coventry. Anaesthesia for shoulder surgery. *Cont Edu Anaesth Crit Care Pain* 2008; **8**(6): 193–8.

P. Kumar, D. M. Coventry. Ultrasound-guided brachial plexus blocks. *Cont Edu Anaesth Crit Care Pain* 2014; **14**(4): 185–91.

Question 7   Facial Trauma

Q	Marking guidance	Mark	Comments
a	• Brisk bleeding • Dyspnoea • Stridor • Drooling • Odynophagia/painful swallowing • Tracheal deviation • Trismus • Subcutaneous emphysema of neck and chest • Voice changes • Burns	Any 6	*Early intubation may be required for issues related to the trauma, such as concurrent head injury and cervical spine injury.*
b	Le Fort I = maxilla fractured from rest of face Le Fort II = maxilla and nasal complex fractured from rest of face Le Fort III = whole mid face dissociates from the skull base and facial bones	1 1 1	*The mobility of the mid face is much greater with Le Fort II and III fractures, and will often also involve mandibular fractures.*
c	• Anterior and posterior nasal packing/Epistat (stating nasal packing is not sufficient) • Manual reduction of fractures • Foley catheter balloon tamponade/Rapid Rhino® • Interventional radiology/embolisation of bleeding artery/external carotid artery • External carotid artery ligation	Any 3	*Profuse bleeding risks airway obstruction, especially in the supine position. It is most commonly as a result of trauma to the facial or maxillary arteries and usually responds to packing or balloon tamponade.*
d	• Nasal endotracheal tube • Submental endotracheal tube • Tracheostomy	Any 2	*Oral endotracheal tubes cannot be used for Le Fort fractures, as dental occlusion must be checked intra-operatively.*

(cont.)

Q	Marking guidance	Mark	Comments
e	Airway considerations: • Throat pack required • Surgical damage of endotracheal tube/cuff • Surgical wiring of endotracheal tube to the maxilla • Post-operative intermaxillary fixation (wiring or elastic bands) may be required • Facial nerve monitoring may be required • Shared airway/difficult intra-operative access to the airway/ increased risk of intra-operative circuit disconnection Blood loss can be extensive: • 2 × wide-bore IV access • Group and save sample Other: • Reflex bradycardia when manipulating the mid face • IV dexamethasone to reduce facial swelling • Antibiotics indicated if wound is contaminated/exposed cartilage	Any 6	*There is always a risk of surgical damage to a nasal endotracheal tube at the posterior nasal space.* *The patient should always have wire cutters/scissors at the bedside.* *A single induction dose of muscle relaxant is acceptable.* *Significant oropharyngeal swelling mandates a critical care admission.*

Suggested reading

M. Morosan, A. Parbhoo, N. Curry. Anaesthesia and common oral and maxilla-facial emergencies. *Contin Edu Anaesth Crit Care Pain* 2012; **12**(5): 257–62.

A. Jose, S. A. Nagori, B. Agarwal, O. Bhutia, A. Roychoudhury. Management of maxillofacial trauma in emergency: an update of challenges and controversies. *J Emerg Trauma Shock* 2016; **9**(2): 73–80.

Question 8   Chronic Liver Disease

Q	Marking guidance	Mark	Comments
a	• Hepatitis B/C • Cytomegalovirus/Epstein-Barr virus • Drug induced, e.g. amiodarone, methotrexate • Autoimmune hepatitis • Primary biliary sclerosis • Primary sclerosing cholangitis • Non-alcoholic steatohepatitis • Haemochromatosis • α-1 antitrypsin deficiency • Wilson's disease • Congestive cardiac failure	Any 4 for 2 marks	
b	Cardiovascular: • Hypotension/reduced systemic vascular resistance • Increased cardiac output • Adrenal insufficiency • Masked coronary artery disease • Cardiomyopathy	Any 2	*Other systemic effects include:* • *Vitamin B1 (thiamine) deficiency risks Wernicke's encephalopathy*
	Respiratory: • Pleural effusion • Diaphragmatic splinting (must specify secondary to ascites) • Porto-pulmonary hypertension • Hepato-pulmonary syndrome • Increased risk of acute respiratory distress syndrome	Any 2	• *Depletion of hepatic and muscle glycogen stores may result in hypoglycaemia* • *Muscle wasting is common due to impaired protein synthesis and malnutrition.*
	Haematological: • Anaemia (gastrointestinal blood loss) • Vitamin K dependent factor coagulopathy • Thrombocytopenia/ hypersplenism	Any 2	*The development of hepatic encephalopathy in patients with chronic liver disease can be precipitated by infection, gastrointestinal haemorrhage, electrolyte or acid–base disturbance,*

(cont.)

Q	Marking guidance	Mark	Comments
	Renal: • Pre-renal failure • Hepato-renal syndrome • Hyperaldosteronism	Any 2	*sedative drugs, hypoglycaemia, hypoxia, hypotension or excessive dietary intake of protein. Alternatively, it may be a sign of gradual progression of the liver disease.*
c	Thiopental: reduced plasma protein binding increases available unbound drug	1	*The pharmacokinetics of suxamethonium may be affected by chronic liver disease. Duration of action is prolonged due to a reduced pseudocholinesterase concentration (rarely clinically significant).*
	Rocuronium: prolonged elimination phase due to degree of hepato-biliary excretion	1	
	Morphine: risk of accumulation secondary to reduced metabolism/ reduced hepatic blood flow and reduced extraction ratio	1	
	Alfentanil: plasma protein binding reduced due to reduced α1-acid glycoprotein concentrations (accept reduced rate of elimination due to increased volume of distribution)	1	*It is usually preferable to choose drugs whose metabolism is not dependent on hepatic function:* • *Atracurium and cisatracurium are metabolised by plasma esterases and Hofmann elimination.* • *Remifentanil is metabolised by tissue and plasma esterases (which are preserved even in patients with severe liver disease).*

Q	Marking guidance	Mark	Comments
d	Option 1: fentanyl PCA Disadvantage: • Can accumulate in higher doses • Constipation increases risk of ammonia accumulation and subsequent encephalopathy Option 2: regional anaesthesia (accept epidural, transverse abdominis plane block) Disadvantage: • Potential for bleeding-related complications, e.g. haematoma	1 Any 1 1 1	*Non-steroidal anti-inflammatory medications are usually avoided due to the risks of gastrointestinal bleeding, platelet dysfunction and nephrotoxicity.* *Paracetamol is sometimes used with caution in this patient group, depending on the aetiology of liver disease.*
e	Child–Pugh class A: 5%–10% Child–Pugh class C: >50% (accept 50%–60%)	1 1	*Child–Pugh class B carries a risk of 20%–30%.* *The Child–Pugh score is made up of five variables:* • *Grade of encephalopathy* • *Ascites* • *Serum bilirubin* • *Serum albumin* • *Prothrombin time* *Each variable scores 1, 2 or 3 depending on degree of severity.* *Total score of 5–6 = Child–Pugh class A* *Total score of 7–9 = Child–Pugh class B* *Total score of >9 = Child–Pugh class C.*

Suggested reading

R. Vaja, L. McNicol, I. Sisley. Anaesthesia for patients with liver disease. *Cont Edu Anaesth Crit Care Pain* 2010; **10**(1): 15–9.

Question 9   Direct Oral Anticoagulants/Antiplatelet Agents

Q	Marking guidance	Mark	Comments
a	Warfarin: antagonises vitamin K epoxide reductase	1	
	Dabigatran: direct thrombin inhibitor	1	
	Rivaroxaban: direct factor Xa inhibitor	1	
	Aspirin: cyclo-oxygenase 1 inhibitor	1	
	Prasugrel: adenosine $P2Y_{12}$ receptor antagonist (accept inhibition of ADP binding)	1	
b	Advantages: • Rapid onset of activity • Short half-lives • Similar or improved efficacy • Fewer drug interactions • Fixed dosing guidelines • No requirement for monitoring	Any 4	*Warfarin remains the most efficacious agent for anticoagulation of patients with metallic heart valves.*
	Disadvantages: • No antidote for most DOACs • No widely available measure of activity • Not licensed for management of anticoagulation for patients with metallic heart valves • Drug interactions • Less clinical experience than warfarin • Renal impairment affects pharmacokinetics	Any 4	
c	• Warfarin: INR ≤1.4	1	*These are the recommendations of the AAGBI, 2013.*
	• Dabigatran: 48–96 hours, depending on renal function	1	
	• Rivaroxaban: 48 hours	1	
	• Aspirin: no need to stop	1	
	• Prasugrel: 7 days	1	

Q	Marking guidance	Mark	Comments
d	• Idarucizumab is a specific monoclonal antibody against dabigatran	1	*Licensed by the National Institute for Health and Care Excellence in 2016.*
	• Dialysis	1	*Two-thirds of the drug is removed during a 2-hour dialysis session.*
	• Prothrombin complex concentrate (PCC)/fresh frozen plasma (FFP)	1	*The dose of PCC/FFP required is uncertain.*

Suggested reading

V. Koenig-Oberhuber, M. Filipovic. New antiplatelet drugs and new oral anticoagulants. *Br J Anaesth* 2016; 117(Suppl. 2): ii74–84.

Association of Anaesthetists of Great Britain and Ireland. Regional anaesthesia and patients with abnormalities of coagulation. 2013. www.aagbi.org/sites/default/files/rapac_2013_web.pdf. (Accessed 8 September 2018).

Question 10 Smoking

Q	Marking guidance	Mark	Comments
a	• Carbon monoxide (CO) has a greater affinity for haemoglobin than O_2 – decreases oxygen carriage	1	*CO has 250 times more affinity for Hb than O_2.*
	• CO shifts the oxyhaemoglobin dissociation curve to the left/ reduces ability of haemoglobin (Hb) to release O_2	1	*CO also inhibits cytochrome oxidase, the enzyme needed for the synthesis of ATP in mitochondria.*
b	• Hypoxaemia • Laryngospasm • Bronchospasm • Retained or thickened secretions • Atelectasis • Infection	Any 5	*Respiratory effects include decreased oxygen carriage, irritable airways, decreased ciliary function, decreased FEV1 and increased closing capacity.*
c	• Stimulates adrenaline release • Activates sympathetic nervous system • Resets aortic and carotid bodies • Increases myocardial contractility • Increases myocardial oxygen demand • Increases heart rate/blood pressure	Any 4	*The half-life of nicotine is approximately 2 hours. Abstinence from smoking on the day of surgery will reduce myocardial demand.*
d	• Anxiety • Withdrawal or agitation • Increased risk of post-operative nausea and vomiting • Airway reactivity • Increased secretions	Any 3	*Smoking cessation in patients with asthma may briefly worsen symptoms and increase airway reactivity.*
e	• Clearance of CO • Improved ciliary function • Nicotine levels return to normal • Reduced myocardial oxygen demand (accept reduction in heart rate)	Any 3	*Quitting 14 days prior to surgery improves airway reactivity and returns sputum levels to normal.*

(cont.)

Q	Marking guidance	Mark	Comments
f	• Polycythaemia • Enhanced platelet function • Increased fibrinogen • Pre-existing vessel disease	Any 3	*This risk is further increased in women taking the oral contraceptive pill.*

Suggested reading

N. Thiagarajan. Smoking and anaesthesia. World Federation of Societies of Anaesthesiologists' Anaesthesia Tutorial of the Week 221. 2011. www.aagbi.org/sites/default/files/221-Smoking-and-Anaesthesia.pdf. (Accessed 26 October 2018).

Question 11 Ultrasound

Q	Marking guidance	Mark	Comments
a	Definition: sound waves of frequency > 20 kHz	1	*Audible limits of human hearing are 20 Hz to 20 kHz.*
	Principles: • Transducer contains material with piezoelectric properties • Piezoelectric material deforms when an alternating electric current is applied • This results in sound wave formation • Sound waves are reflected back at tissue interfaces • Difference in tissue density at interfaces will determine degree of reflection • Sounds reflected to the transducer are amplified and converted to an image	Any 5	*There are many types of ultrasound used:* • *'A' mode = amplitude* • *'B' mode = brightness* • *'M' mode = motion*
b	• Gain: increasing the gain amplifies the overall signal • Higher frequency improves resolution at the expense of penetration; lower frequency permits deeper penetration	1 1	*The proportion of sound waves beam reflected to the transducer can be altered through small changes to the angle of the transducer. 'Rocking' the ultrasound probe is used to improve the image of structures: this is known as anisotropy.*

Q	Marking guidance	Mark	Comments
c	• Acoustic enhancement → more sound energy passes through fluid filled structures, enhancing the tissues behind these structures	6	*E.g. ultrasound of gynaecological structures behind an intentionally full bladder.*
	• Acoustic shadowing → when sound energy hits a highly reflective structure, tissues behind this structure appear dark		
	• Reverberation → ultrasound pulse becomes 'caught' between two parallel surfaces and reverberates between them causing a repetitive artefact on the image		*'Comet tails' on lung ultrasound are an example of reverberation. The loss of comet tails is abnormal and seen in pneumothorax.*
	• Refraction → as ultrasound travels through different mediums, a change in velocity can alter its direction		*One mark per artefact, and 1 mark for each correct explanation*
d	Left ventricular outflow tract (LVOT) area	1	$SV = LVOT\ area \times VTI$
	Velocity time integral (VTI)	1	$CO = SV \times HR$
e	• Venous/arterial cannulation	Any 4	
	• Lung imaging: pneumothorax/ pleural effusions		
	• Locating neck vessels prior to tracheostomy		
	• Regional anaesthesia		
	• Cardiac output monitoring		
	• Epidural space location		
	• Transcranial Doppler		

Suggested reading

M. MacGregor, L. Kelliher, J. Kirk-Bayley. The physics of ultrasound part 1. World Federation of Societies of Anaesthesiologists' Anaesthesia Tutorial of the Week 199. 2010. www.aagbi.org/sites/default/files/199-The-physics-of-ultrasound-part-1.pdf. (Accessed 26 October 2018).

M. MacGregor, L. Kelliher, J. Kirk-Bayley. The physics of ultrasound part 2. World Federation of Societies of Anaesthesiologists' Anaesthesia Tutorial of the Week 218, 2011. www.aagbi.org/sites/default/files/218-The-Physics-of-Ultrasound-part-2.pdf. (Accessed 26 October 2018).

Question 12 Cataract

	Marking guidance	Mark	Comments
a	• Reduced risk of nosocomial infection • Earlier return to normal activity and mobilisation • Reduced anxiety if overnight stay avoided • Reduction in venous thromboembolic events • Recovery at home • Increased patient satisfaction	Any 3	*The British Association of Day Surgery publishes targets for day and short-stay surgery for more than 200 different procedures.*
b	• Reduced waiting times • Value for money and reduced cost to hospital • Best practice tariff • Quicker turnover of patients • Possible reduction of post-operative complications • Lower risk of cancellation • Overnight beds spared for major surgical cases • More efficient theatre utilisation	Any 3	
c	• Patients must understand, engage with and consent to the surgical procedure • There must be a responsible person to escort the patient home and remain with them for 24 hours • Home circumstances suitable for post-operative care • Access to a telephone • Geographical proximity to hospital/transport time < 1 hour • Toilet facilities and central heating required in some geographical locations	Any 3	*Some units employ carers to stay with a post-operative patient overnight if they live alone, as this is more cost-effective than an overnight hospital stay.*

(cont.)

	Marking guidance	Mark	Comments
d	Continue warfarin at usual dose: anticoagulation should not be stopped	1	*Anticoagulants and antiplatelet agents should be continued in the perioperative period for patients undergoing cataract operations as day patient surgery. Normal therapeutic targets should be maintained, as the risk of bleeding is outweighed by the increased risk of significant thrombotic events.*
e	• Stop before you block	1	
	• Apply topical anaesthesia to the eye	Any 5	*E.g. amethocaine 0.5% or 1%.*
	• Aqueous sterilising solution		*E.g. povidone-iodine 5% aqueous solution.*
	• Barraquer lid speculum		
	• Ask the patient to look 'up and out' to expose the infranasal quadrant		
	• Use non-toothed (Moorfields) forceps to lift the conjunctiva and Tenon's fascia 5–10 mm from the limbus		
	• Make a small cut with Westcott scissors to expose the underlying scleral layer		
	• Carefully make a passage with Westcott scissors		
	• Attach a blunt ended sub-Tenon's cannula to a syringe containing local anaesthetic and advance this along the passage following the contour of the eyeball until the syringe is vertical		

(cont.)

	Marking guidance	Mark	Comments
	• Aspirate then inject the local anaesthetic		*E.g. 3–5 mL of a 50:50 solution containing 2% lignocaine and 0.5% bupivacaine.*
f	• Chemosis • Sub-conjunctival haemorrhage • Pain • Ecchymoses • Retro-bulbar haemorrhage • Globe injury • Optic nerve atrophy • Muscular palsy • Brainstem anaesthesia	Any 4	*Globe perforation, retro-bulbar haemorrhage and optic nerve damage all have approximately 1% incidence.*

Further reading

D. J. Quemby, M. E. Stocker. Day surgery development and practice: key factors for a successful pathway. *Cont Edu Anaesth Crit Care Pain* 2014; **14**(6): 256–61.

R. Anker, N. Kaur. Regional anaesthesia for ophthalmic surgery. *BJA Educ* 2017; **17**(7): 221–7.

Paper 9 Answers

Question 1   Myotonic Dystrophy

Q	Marking guidance	Mark	Comments
a	• Myotonic dystrophy = multisystem genetic condition characterised by muscle weakness/loss	1	*There are two main types of myotonic dystrophy: DM1 due to mutation of the DMPK gene, and DM2 due to mutation of the CNBP gene.*
	• Pathophysiology: abnormal Na^+ or Cl^- channels, which results in impaired muscle relaxation	1	
	• Inheritance: autosomal dominant	1	
b	• Frontal balding • Characteristic weakness/ wasting of: – Facial muscles – Levator palpebrae → bilateral ptosis – Muscles of mastication – Sternocleidomastoid	Any 2	*The characteristic facial appearance is described as a 'myopathic' or 'hatchet' appearance.*
c	Respiratory: • Respiratory muscle weakness • Restrictive lung disease • Poor cough • Central and obstructive sleep apnoea	Any 2	*Myotonic dystrophy is a multisystem disease with many implications for anaesthetists.*
	Cardiovascular: • Cardiac conduction defects/ heart block • Cardiomyopathy/congestive heart failure	Any 2	
	Central nervous system: • Behavioural problems/ cognitive decline • Central hypersomnia • Susceptibility to sedatives/ analgesics	Any 1	

Q	Marking guidance	Mark	Comments
	Gastrointestinal: • Bulbar weakness/swallowing difficulty • Delayed gastric emptying	Any 1	
	Endocrine: • Thyroid/adrenal impairment • Testicular atrophy • Type II diabetes mellitus	Any 1	
d	• Bulbar palsy mandates intubation • Risk of aspiration pneumonia is high – consider prokinetics, antacids and rapid sequence induction • Awake arterial line (given significant cardiovascular disease) • Judicious use of intravenous induction agent due to risk of cardiorespiratory depression • Intubation and maintenance of anaesthesia can be achieved without use of muscle relaxants • Avoid suxamethonium – may trigger a myotonic contracture • Avoid neuromuscular monitoring – may trigger myotonic contraction	Any 4	*Caution with benzodiazepine pre-medication, as these patients are particularly susceptible to these agents.*

(cont.)

Q	Marking guidance	Mark	Comments
e	• Avoid hypothermia/shivering: may precipitate myotonic contracture • Apply defibrillator/pacer pads: high risk of intra-operative arrhythmias • Avoid nerve stimulator: may precipitate myotonic contraction • Reversal of neuromuscular blockade: neostigmine may precipitate myotonic contraction • Multimodal analgesia/ judicious use of systemic opioids • Blood glucose monitoring, as diabetes is common in myotonic dystrophy	Any 4	

Suggested reading

S. Marsh, A. Pittard. Neuromuscular disorders and anaesthesia. Part 2: specific neuromuscular disorders. *Cont Edu Anaesth Crit Care Pain* 2011; **11**(4): 119–23.

Question 2 Cardiac Implantable Devices

Q	Marking guidance	Mark	Comments
a	Letter 1: chamber paced Letter 2: chamber sensed Letter 3: mode of response/ response to sensing Letter 4: programmability/rate modulation Letter 5: multi-site function	5	*Implantable cardioverter defibrillators (ICDs) have a four-letter coding system:* • *Letter 1 = chamber shocked* • *Letter 2 = chamber paced during anti-tachycardia functions* • *Letter 3 = method through which tachycardia is detected* • *Letter 4 = chambers paced during anti-bradycardia functions*
b	Minimum intrinsic atrial or ventricular electrical activity that is sensed by the device (measured in mV)	1	*If incorrectly set, the device may fail to detect intrinsic atrial or ventricular activity. This can result in* • *Over-pacing – firing despite intrinsic activity, which risks triggering malignant tachyarrhythmias.* • *Under-sensing – which leads to a failure to pace despite there being no intrinsic electrical activity.*
c	• ECG	1	*ECG may demonstrate pacing activity:* • *Atrial pacing = spike followed by a P-wave* • *Ventricular pacing = spike followed by a broad QRS complex.*
	• Chest X-ray	1	*Chest X-ray shows the number and configuration*

(cont.)

Q	Marking guidance	Mark	Comments
			of leads, and may also demonstrate lead fracture or migration.
	• Electrolytes	1	*Electrolyte abnormalities (especially of potassium and magnesium) may precipitate arrhythmias and/or interfere with pacemaker capture.*
d	• Any patient with significant permanent pacemaker (PPM) dependency	1	*If there is the potential for electromagnetic interference during the procedure, temporary re-programming of the PPM to an asynchronous (non-sensing) mode (e.g. AOO, VOO or DOO) may be required.*
	• Any PPM with rate-responsive functions	1	*Otherwise mechanical ventilation may stimulate excessive pacing rates.*
	• Any defibrillator function	1	*Electromagnetic interference during the procedure may trigger inappropriate defibrillation. If deactivation is not possible (e.g. emergency surgery), the application of a magnet may be considered.*
e	Devices: • Medical equipment incorporating wireless technology • Mobile phones	Any 4	*Diathermy should be avoided where possible; bipolar is considered safer than monopolar. If monopolar diathermy is*

(cont.)

Q	Marking guidance	Mark	Comments
	Procedures: • Radiofrequency ablation • Insertion of tissue expanders • Electroconvulsive therapy • Transcutaneous electric nerve stimulation • Radiation therapy • Extracorporeal shock-wave lithotripsy		*absolutely necessary, short 1–2 s bursts with 10 s pauses should be used, and cutting current is safer than coagulation current.* *The pathway from the diathermy to the ground electrode should not pass near the CIED.*
f	PPM: asynchronous mode/fixed rate pacing	1	*Less commonly, application of a magnet to a PPM initiates a diagnostics function, followed by reversion to its programmed mode of pacing.*
	ICD: deactivation of shock and anti-tachycardia pacing functions	1	*Magnet application has no effect on bradycardia pacing of ICDs.*
g	10–15 cm	1	*Anterior–posterior pad placement is usually preferred.*
h	Damage to the myocardium as a consequence of excess current flow	1	

Suggested reading

H. Bryant, P. Diprose. Perioperative management of patients with cardiac implantable electronic devices. *Cont Edu Anaesth Crit Care Pain* 2016; **16**(11): 388–96.

R Pervez. Pacemakers and Implantable Cardioverter-Defibrillators. World Federation of Societies of Anaesthesiologists' Anaesthesia Tutorial of the Week 299. 2013. www.aagbi.org/sites/default/files/299%20Pacemakers%20and%20ICDs%20Part%201.pdf. (Accessed 5 September 2018).

Question 3   Pancreatitis

Q	Marking guidance	Mark	Comments
a	• Exocrine function: secretion of pancreatic juice (bicarbonate, electrolytes and proteolytic enzymes) • Endocrine function: secretion of insulin, glucagon, somatostatin	2	*Approximately 1500 mL of pancreatic juice is secreted per day.*
b	• Vomiting • Pyrexia • Abdominal distension • Peritonism • Grey–Turner's sign: discolouration of the flanks • Cullen's sign: peri-umbilical discolouration • Fox's sign: discolouration of the inguinal ligament	Any 4	*The classical signs are a result of retroperitoneal haemorrhage tracking along tissue planes.*
c	Obstructive: • Gallstones • Neoplasm/metastasis • Chronic alcohol abuse • Cystic fibrosis Parenchymal: • Trauma (blunt or penetrating) • Following endoscopic retrograde cholangiopancreatography Global: • Hypoxia/systemic inflammatory response syndrome/sepsis Toxic: • Acute alcohol intake • Drugs (azathioprine, non-steroidal anti-inflammatory drugs, diuretics) • Hypothermia • Hypercalcaemia Other: • Idiopathic	Any 5	Not acceptable: scorpion bites, a rare cause of pancreatitis.

Q	Marking guidance	Mark	Comments
d	General factors: • Age 70 years or older • Body mass index over 30 kg/m^2 Indicators of more severe disease: • Not responsive to fluid resuscitation • >30% necrosis of the pancreas • Pleural effusions • Three or more of Ranson's criteria • CRP > 150 mg/L at 48 hours	Any 4	Ranson's criteria is a scoring system to predict acute pancreatitis and associated mortality. It is scored on admission and at 48 hours. The factors taken into account are • White cell count • Lactate dehydrogenase • Aspartate transaminase • Age > 55 years • Glucose • Serum calcium • Haematocrit • Arterial partial pressure of oxygen • Urea • Base deficit • Fluid deficit
e	• Relieving biliary obstruction (e.g. ERCP) • Removing infected intra- and extra-pancreatic necrosis	2	Necrosectomy carries a high mortality.
f	Within 72 hours	1	According to NICE guideline 104.
g	• Cheaper • Safer • Avoids need for central line • Associated with fewer complications • Better outcome overall	3	

Suggested reading

S. P. Young, J. P. Thompson. Severe acute pancreatitis. *Cont Edu Anaesth Crit Care Pain* 2008; 8(4): 125–8.

National Institute for Health and Care Excellence. Pancreatitis: diagnosis and management NG 104. 2018. www .nice.org.uk/guidance/ng104/documents/ draft-guideline. (Accessed 16 November 2018).

Question 4 Tracheoesophageal Fistula

Q	Marking guidance	Mark	Comments
a	1 in 3000 live births (accept 1:3000 to 1:5000)	1	
b	• Cardiac • Vertebral • Anorectal • Urogenital • Laryngo-tracheal/palatal • Skeletal/limb • Gastrointestinal • Renal	Any 3	TOF is associated with the following syndromes/ chromosomal abnormalities: • Holt–Oram syndrome • DiGeorge syndrome • Polysplenia • Pierre–Robin syndrome • Trisomy 18 • Trisomy 21
c	• Avoiding bag–mask ventilation • Gaseous induction • Suction/aspiration of upper oesophageal pouch • Topicalisation of airway • Intubation under inhalational anaesthesia • Maintenance of spontaneous ventilation • Use of flexible bronchoscope to ensure positioning of tracheal tube beyond fistula site • Use of muscle relaxant only once tracheal tube is correctly positioned	Any 3	Before induction of anaesthesia, the upper pouch tube is aspirated and then removed. Bag–mask ventilation is avoided to prevent problematic gastric inflation. A rigid bronchoscopic examination of the trachea and main bronchi is performed to confirm the position of the TOF. The tracheal tube is then positioned such that it occludes the TOF. Only once the tracheal tube has been correctly positioned is a muscle relaxant given.
d	Respiratory: • Ventilation is primarily diaphragmatic • Diaphragm easily splinted by abdominal organ content • Lower functional residual capacity (FRC)	Any 3	Neonatal airway differences include • Large head, short neck and a prominent occiput • Large tongue • High and anterior larynx, at the level of C3/4

358

Q	Marking guidance	Mark	Comments
	• Rate dependent minute ventilation/unable to increase tidal volume • Closing volume > FRC/greater risk of airway collapse • Respiratory muscles easily fatigued • Lower number of alveoli		*• Long, U-shaped epiglottis that flops posteriorly* *• Neonates are obligate nasal breathers* *• Airway is funnel shaped and narrowest at the level of the cricoid cartilage*
	Cardiovascular: • Cardiac output is rate dependent/fixed cardiac output • Less compliant myocardium • Dominant parasympathetic tone/tendency towards bradycardia • Higher blood volume per kg than adults • Transitional circulation	Any 3	*The ductus arteriosus contracts in the first few days of life and normally fibroses within 2–4 weeks. Foramen ovale closure usually occurs in the first day of life.* *In response to hypoxia and acidosis, reversion to the transitional circulation may occur in the first few weeks after birth.*
	Haematological: • Significant proportion of haemoglobin is of foetal HbF type • Higher haematocrit/red cell mass • Oxyhaemoglobin disassociation curve shifted to the left • Deficient platelet function • Deficiency of vitamin K dependent clotting factors	Any 3	*At birth, HbF comprises 70%–90% of Hb. At 3 months, HbF comprises only 5%.* *Typical newborn Hb is 180–200 g/L (haematocrit ~0.6).*

(cont.)

Q	Marking guidance	Mark	Comments
e	• High surface area to volume ratio • Minimal subcutaneous tissue • Poorly developed shivering • Poor vasoconstrictive capabilities • Brown fat metabolism for thermogenesis requires significant amounts of oxygen	Any 3	*Hypothermia in neonates causes respiratory depression, acidosis, decreased cardiac output, increases the duration of action of drugs, decreases platelet function and increases the risk of infection.*
f	40–60 mL/kg	1	*24-hour fluid requirements in the first days of life are dependent on weight and degree of prematurity. For full-term neonates ≥ 2.0 kg, the first 5 days' fluid requirements are* • *Day 1: 40–60 mL/kg/24 hours* • *Day 2: 60–90 mL/kg/24 hours* • *Day 3: 80–100 mL/kg/24 hours* • *Day 4: 100–120 mL/kg/24 hours* • *Day 5: 120–150 mL/kg/24 hours*

Suggested reading

F. Macfarlane. Paediatric anatomy and physiology and the basics of paediatric anaesthesia. World Federation of Societies of Anaesthesiologists' Anaesthesia Tutorial of the Week 7, 2005. www.aagbi.org/sites/default/files/7-Paediatric-anatomy-physiology-and-the-basics-of-paediatric-anaesthesia.pdf. (Accessed 29 September 2018).

O. Al-Rawi, P.D. Booker. Oesophageal atresia and tracheo-oesophageal fistula. *Cont Edu Anaesth Crit Care Pain* 2007, 7(1): 15–9.

Question 5   Placenta

Q	Marking guidance	Mark	Comments
a	• Gas exchange • Nutrient and waste transfer • Transfer of immunity • Hormone secretion • Barrier function	Any 3	*The placenta is the sole physical link between mother and foetus, with a surface area of almost 15 m².*
b	• Simple diffusion • Facilitated diffusion • Active transport • Pinocytosis	4	*E.g. midazolam, paracetamol* *E.g. cephalosporins* *E.g. noradrenaline*
c	• Placental surface area • Placental thickness • pH of maternal/foetal blood • Placental metabolism • Uteroplacental blood flow • Presence of drug transporters • Molecular weight of drug • Lipid solubility • pKa of drug • Protein binding • Concentration gradient	Any 6	*Drugs with a molecular weight < 500 Da readily diffuse across placenta. Only the unionised fraction of the drug crosses the placental membrane. Drugs that are protein-bound do not diffuse across the placenta.*
d	• Systemic absorption • Highly lipid soluble, crosses placenta to foetus by simple diffusion • Decreased foetal pH results in increased ionised fraction of drug • Ionised form less able to cross placenta back into maternal circulation	Any 4	*Bupivacaine and ropivacaine are highly lipid soluble but have a high degree of protein binding, limiting placental transfer.* *Lignocaine is less lipid soluble but a lower degree of protein binding accounts for its higher relative foetal blood level.*

(cont.)

Q	Marking guidance	Mark	Comments
e	Potential adverse effect: • Bradycardia • Neostigmine is a small molecule and crosses placenta/ glycopyrrolate is fully ionised therefore does not cross placenta	2	*Although neostigmine is a quaternary ammonium compound, it has a small molecular weight, crossing the placenta more rapidly than glycopyrrolate.*
	Mitigate by: • Can use atropine instead of glycopyrrolate	1	*Atropine is a lipid soluble tertiary amine which crosses the placenta easily.*

Suggested reading

S. K. Griffiths, J. P. Campbell. Placental structure, function and drug transfer. *Cont Edu Anaesth Crit Care Pain* 2015; **15**(2): 84–9.

Question 6 Labour Analgesia

Q	Marking guidance	Mark	Comments
a	<u>Visceral pain</u> • Uterine contraction and cervical dilatation • Unmyelinated C-fibres • Travel with sympathetic fibres through uterine and cervical plexuses • T10–L1 nerve roots	Any 3	*Chemical mediators involved include bradykinin, leukotrienes, prostaglandins, serotonin, substance P and lactic acid.* *Transmission to the hypothalamic and limbic systems accounts for the emotional and autonomic responses associated with pain.*
	<u>Somatic pain</u> • Perineal, pelvic floor and vaginal stretching or injury • A-δ fibres • Via pudendal nerves • S2–S4 nerve roots • Also via ilioinguinal nerves/genitofemoral nerves to L1/2	Any 3	*Somatic pain occurs closer to delivery and is more resistant to opioid analgesia.*
b	Anterior: posterior longitudinal ligament (accept vertebral bodies/intervertebral discs) Posterior: ligamentum flavum Superior: foramen magnum Inferior: sacrococcygeal membrane	4	*Lateral boundaries: pedicles and intervertebral foraminae.* *The contents of the epidural space include fat, dural sac, spinal nerves, vessels and connective tissue.*
c	• Cross the dura • Bind to opioid receptors in spinal cord white matter/dorsal horns/substantia gelatinosa • Systemic absorption from epidural veins • Cephalic spread and brainstem action	Any 3	*Stimulation of opioid receptors closes calcium channels, resulting in potassium efflux and reduced cAMP production, which then results in reduced neuronal cell excitability.*

(cont.)

Q	Marking guidance	Mark	Comments
d	• Rapid onset of action • Shorter duration of action • Minimal cephalad spread reducing risk of respiratory depression	1 1 1	*Diamorphine crosses the dura more rapidly than morphine but slower than fentanyl.*
e	Grade 2: free movement of feet, just able to flex knees Grade 3: free movement of feet, unable to flex knees	1 1	
f	<u>Steps:</u> • Stop the infusion • Reassess every 30 min <u>Request MRI scan:</u> If no improvement in leg strength and 4 hours have elapsed since stopping the epidural	Any 1 1	*An epidural haematoma should be suspected if leg strength does not improve. Earlier neurosurgical referral should be considered if you do not have access to MRI.* *An epidural haematoma must be evacuated within 8 hours of symptom onset for the best chance of recovery.*

Suggested reading

S. Labor, S. Maguire. The pain of labour. *Rev Pain* 2008; **2**: 15–9.

E. McGrady, K. Litchfield. Epidural analgesia in labour. *Cont Edu Anaesth Crit Care Pain* 2004; **4**: 114–7.

Association of Anaesthetists of Great Britain and Ireland. Best practice in the management of epidural analgesia in the hospital setting, 2010. www.aagbi.org/sites/default/files/epidural_analgesia_2011.pdf. (Accessed 27 October 2018).

Question 7 Transurethral Resection Syndrome

Q	Marking guidance	Mark	Comments
a	• Early detection of complications • Reduced blood loss • Post-operative analgesia • Reduced incidence of venous thromboembolism	4	*Complications such as transurethral resection (TUR) syndrome and bladder perforation are detected earlier under regional anaesthesia.*
b	Sympathetic: T11–L2 Parasympathetic: S2–S4	1 1	*Via the pelvic (inferior hypogastric) plexus.*
c	Block height: T10 Reason: to eliminate the discomfort from bladder distension	1	Both parts must be correct for 1 mark
d	• Transparent • Non-conductive • Isotonic • Non-toxic • Non-haemolytic • Easy to sterilise • Cheap	Any 4	*The most commonly used irrigation fluid in the UK is glycine 1.5%, which is hypotonic (osmolalilty of 220 mOsmol/kg).*
e	• Pressure of irrigation fluid/ height of irrigation bag • Low venous pressure/ hypovolaemia • Prolonged surgery • Significant blood loss/open veins • Capsular/bladder perforation	Any 4	*Capsular or bladder perforation allows a large volume of irrigation fluid into the peritoneal cavity, where it is rapidly absorbed.*
f	Stop surgery	1	

(cont.)

Q	Marking guidance	Mark	Comments
g	Clinical feature: Circulatory overload/pulmonary oedema/cardiac failure	1	
	Pathophysiology: Due to excessive absorption of irrigation solution	1	
	Clinical feature: Agitation/nausea/seizures/coma	1	
	Pathophysiology: Hypo-osmolality/hyponatraemia secondary to dilutional effect of absorbing hypo-osmolar irrigation fluid	1	*Hypo-osmolality is more important than hyponatraemia in CNS disturbance.*
	Clinical feature: Nausea/headache/weakness/visual disturbances (including transient blindness)	1	
	Pathophysiology: Glycine toxicity	1	*Glycine is a major inhibitory neurotransmitter in the CNS and retina.*

Suggested reading

A. M. O'Donnell, I. Foo. Anaesthesia for transurethral resection of the prostate. *Cont Edu Anaesth Crit Care Pain* 2009; **9**(3): 92–6.

Question 8 Fat Embolus

Q	Marking guidance	Mark	Comments
a	• Respiratory system	1	*Most commonly dyspnoea, tachypnoea and hypoxaemia.*
	• Central nervous system	1	*Transient neurological features result from cerebral embolism, with a spectrum from mild confusion and drowsiness through to seizures.*
	• Skin	1	*A petechial rash is often the last component of the triad to develop, occurring in 60% of cases. It is caused by embolisation of small dermal capillaries leading to extravasation of erythrocytes. This most commonly takes place in the conjunctiva, oral mucous membrane and skin folds of the upper body, especially the neck and axilla.*
b	• Pyrexia > 38.5°C • Tachycardia > 110 beats/min • Myocardial ischaemia • Emboli present on fundoscopy • A sudden inexplicable drop in haematocrit or platelets • Increasing ESR • Lipouria • Fat globules present in the sputum	Any 3	*At least one major and four minor of Gurd's diagnostic criteria must be present for a diagnosis of fat embolism to be made. Alternative diagnostic methods are Lindeque's criteria and Schonfeld's criteria.*

(cont.)

Q	Marking guidance	Mark	Comments
c	<u>Theory 1:</u> mechanical Mechanism:	1	*Whilst the mechanical theory is supported by the echogenic observation of material passing into the right heart during orthopaedic surgery, it does not sufficiently explain the 24- to 48-hour delay in symptom onset that is usually seen.*
	• Fat from disrupted bone marrow enters venules	1	
	• Subsequently able to enter venous circulation and embolise in pulmonary circulation	1	
	<u>Theory 2:</u> biochemical/toxic intermediaries Mechanism:	1	*The biochemical theory may better explain the delay in onset of symptoms in fat embolism syndrome because of the timescale required to produce toxic metabolites.*
	• Embolised fat agglutinates/degrades in plasma	1	
	• Results in production of potentially toxic metabolites such as free fatty acids/chylomicrons which damage capillary beds	1	
d	• Pelvic fractures • Fractures of other marrow-containing bones • Orthopaedic procedures • Soft tissue injuries • Burns	Any 2	
e	• Bone marrow harvesting and transplant • Pancreatitis • Diabetes mellitus • Osteomyelitis and panniculitis • Bone tumour lysis • Steroid therapy • Sickle cell haemoglobinopathies • Alcoholic (fatty) liver disease • Lipid fusion • Total parenteral nutrition	Any 2	

Q	Marking guidance	Mark	Comments
f	• Early immobilisation • Early surgical fixation • Use of venting holes intra-operatively • Avoiding intra-medullary nailing	Any 2	*Management is supportive:* • *Immobilise fracture* • *Optimise oxygenation* • *Lung-protective ventilation* • *Avoid hypovolaemia* • *DVT and peptic ulcer prophylaxis* *Therapies that have been suggested but are considered ineffective include steroids, heparin, alcohol and dextran.*
g	Anaemia Thrombocytopenia	Any 1	*Raised ESR and hypofibrinogenaemia are also commonly seen.*
h	5%–15%	1	

Suggested reading

A. Gupta, C. Reilly. Fat embolism. *Cont Edu Anaesth Crit Care Pain* 2007; 7(5): 148–51.

Question 9   Nitrous Oxide

Q	Marking guidance	Mark	Comments
a	• Induction and maintenance of anaesthesia, in combination with a volatile agent • To provide a rapid onset and offset of anaesthesia/second gas effect with volatile agent • Obstetrics and labour analgesia/supplementation in theatre as Entonox • Analgesia (pre-hospital, Emergency Department, burns dressing changes, orthopaedic manipulation)	Any 3	
b	Molecular weight: 44 g/mol Boiling point: 36.5°C (accept 35°–38°C) Minimum alveolar concentration: 105%	1 1 1	
c	• Commercially produced by heating ammonium nitrate to 170°–240°C • $NH_4NO_3 \rightarrow N_2O + 2H_2O$ • Stored in French blue cylinders at 4400 kPa (4.4 bar) and room temperature • N_2O is stored as a liquid and vapour/stored below critical temperature	4	*By-products such as nitrogen (N_2), nitrogen dioxide (NO_2) and nitric acid (HNO_3) are removed by scrubbing agents and base/acid gas washes.*
d	<u>Respiratory system:</u> • Decreased tidal volume but increased respiratory rate, hence minute volume usually maintained • Hypoxic pulmonary vasoconstriction impaired at high N_2O concentration	Any 2	*N_2O does not cause bronchodilation, unlike the halogenated volatile anaesthetic agents.*

Q	Marking guidance	Mark	Comments
	• Depressed mucociliary flow/ neutrophil chemotaxis therefore may increase post-op respiratory complications		
	Cardiovascular system:	Any 2	
	• Direct myocardial depression: mild negative inotropic effect		*Overall, cardiac output is usually maintained.*
	• Increased sympathetic outflow		
	• Increased pulmonary vascular resistance due to constriction of pulmonary vascular smooth muscle		*Therefore right atrial pressure may increase.*
e	• Increased incidence of post-operative nausea and vomiting	Any 6	
	• Diffusion hypoxia during washout phase		
	• Expansion of air-filled spaces, e.g. intestine, middle ear, pneumothorax/bullae		
	• May cause/exacerbate air embolism/pneumocephalus/ raised intraocular pressure when using intraocular gas		
	• Prolonged administration can lead to complete bone marrow failure/megaloblastic changes		*>12 hour administration*
	• B_{12} oxidation may result in paraesthesia/subacute combined cord degeneration		
	• Potential for teratogenicity		*Evidence in animal models.*
	• Potential minor contributor as greenhouse gas		
	• Potential to administer hypoxic mixture		*Anaesthetic machines have safety features to prevent this.*

Suggested reading

S. M. Brown, J. R. Sneyd. Nitrous oxide in
modern anaesthetic practice. *BJA Educ*
2016; **16**(3): 87–91.

Question 10 Substance Abuse

Q	Marking guidance	Mark	Comments
a	Repeated, excessive or inappropriate use of a mood-altering substance resulting in negative consequences	1	*This definition encompasses all substances including alcohol abuse.*
b	Dependence: a state of physical adaptation which leads to withdrawal symptoms upon cessation of drug use	1	*Addiction is characterised by impaired control over drug use despite harm. It is a primary, chronic, neurobiological disease which is multifactorial in nature. The rate of onset of addiction is directly related to the potency of the drug abused.*
	Tolerance: state of adaptation in which exposure to a drug induces changes that result in diminution of its effects over time	1	
c	• Opioids • Alcohol • Marijuana • Cocaine • Midazolam	Any 3	*Intravenous opioids are the most commonly abused drugs. Anaesthetic agents including propofol and inhalational agents can also be abused.*
d	General risk factors: • Parental history of substance abuse • Childhood abuse • Dysfunctional family • Mental health disorder • Male sex • History of experimenting with drugs • Peers who use drugs	Any 4	*Drug abuse as a medical student may lead to trainees entering specialties where there is easier access to drugs.*
	Specific to doctors: • Occupational access to controlled substances • Long hours • High stress • Practising in anaesthesia, emergency medicine, psychiatry, academic medicine • Self-prescription	Any 3	

(cont.)

Q	Marking guidance	Mark	Comments
e	• Harm to patient • Harm to self/suicide risk • Financial risk (accept payment for illicit drugs) • Social consequences, e.g. breakdown of relationships • Prosecution may result in loss of job	Any 3	
f	Definition: return to substance use after a period of abstinence Predictors: • History of relapse • Family history of substance abuse • Mental health disorder • Intravenous opioid use	1 Any 3	

Suggested reading

R. M. Mayall. Substance abuse in anaesthetists. *BJA Educ* 2016; **16**(7): 236–41.

Question 11   Cardiac Output Monitoring

Q	Marking guidance	Mark	Comments
a	Swan–Ganz catheter (accept thermodilution catheter)	1	*Despite the decline in the use of the Swan–Ganz catheter, it is still considered the gold standard for cardiac output measurement against which all new monitors are measured.*
b	• Marker of oxygen delivery to tissues • Guides fluid resuscitation • Guides use of vasoactive and/or inotropic medications	Any 2	
c	Preload: end-diastolic ventricular wall tension (accept tension at the point of maximal filling) Afterload: tension developed in the ventricular wall during systole (accept tension generated in order to eject blood during systole) Mean arterial pressure (MAP): average arterial blood pressure throughout the cardiac cycle (accept correct equation as definition: MAP = diastolic BP + 1/3 pulse pressure)	1 1 1	*Preload is mainly determined by right ventricular filling.* *Afterload is usually determined by systemic vascular resistance, although it is also affected by ventricular volume, wall thickness and conditions that may obstruct outflow (e.g. aortic stenosis).*
d	Doppler effect: apparent change in received frequency due to relative motion between a sound source and sound receiver	1	

(cont.)

Q	Marking guidance	Mark	Comments
e	• Ultrasound waves generated by the transducer are reflected back to it from moving red blood cells	1	*Doppler equation:* $$V = \frac{F_d c}{2 F_o \cos \theta}$$ *where F_0 is the transmitted Doppler frequency, F_d is the change in frequency (Doppler shift), V is the velocity of blood in the descending thoracic aorta, θ is the beam angle and c is the speed of sound in tissue.*
	• The resultant Doppler shift is used to determine the velocity of blood in the descending thoracic aorta	1	
	• The cross-sectional surface area of the aorta is estimated from a nomogram based on the height, weight and age of the patient	1	
	• The velocity and the cross-sectional area are multiplied together to determine flow	1	
	• A correction factor is made to account for the fact that only ~70% of cardiac output transits the descending thoracic aorta	1	
f	Flow time corrected:		*A low FTc may indicate hypovolaemia or increased afterload. A high FTc may be seen in patients with low afterload.*
	• Definition: duration of flow during systole, corrected for heart rate	1	
	• Normal value: 330–360 ms	1	
	Peak velocity:		*Typical peak velocity values drop with age:*
	• Definition: highest blood velocity detected during systole	1	*• 70–100 cm/s at 50 years*
	• Normal value: 70–120 cm/s	1	*• 50–80 cm/s at 80 years* *Peak velocity is used as a surrogate of left ventricular contractility.*

(cont.)

Q	Marking guidance	Mark	Comments
g	• May require sedation/limited use in awake patients • User dependent • Interference from surgical instruments, e.g. diathermy • Depends on accurate probe positioning • Probe may detect other vessels, e.g. intracardiac/intrapulmonary • Assumes a constant percentage of cardiac output (~70%) enters the descending thoracic aorta • Nomogram based on population data, which may be inaccurate	Any 4	

Suggested reading

T. Lawson. Cardiac output monitoring part 1. World Federation of Societies of Anaesthesiologists' Anaesthesia Tutorial of the Week 183, 2010. www.frca.co.uk/Documents/183%20Cardiac%20output%20monitoring%20-%20part%201.pdf. (Accessed 8 October 2018).

K. Drummond, E. Murphy. Minimally invasive cardiac output monitors. *Cont Edu Anaesth, Crit Care Pain* 2012; **12**(1): 5–10.

Question 12 Point-of-Care Coagulation Testing

Q	Marking guidance	Mark	Comments
a	Advantages: • Faster time to results compared to laboratory testing • Reduces unnecessary transfusion of blood products • Provides additional information on platelet function and fibrinolysis when compared to laboratory testing • Small volume of blood required • Easy to train staff • Test of in vivo rather than in vitro coagulation	Any 3	
	Disadvantages: • Training of staff members required (to run test and interpret results) • Expensive investment • Must be tested within a short period of time as whole blood is used • Standardised temperature of 37°C hinders detection of coagulopathy secondary to hypothermia • Cannot detect coagulopathies secondary to hypocalcaemia • Significant difference in normal ranges between adults, children and neonates	Any 3	
b	i) Time taken from the start of the test to initial fibrin formation/ concentration of soluble clotting factors in the plasma	1	
	ii) Rapidity of fibrin build up and cross linking/rate of clot formation	1	
	iii) Strength of fibrin clot/	1	

(cont.)

Q	Marking guidance	Mark	Comments
	maximum clot strength/total number and function of platelets and fibrinogen concentration		
	iv) Time to full clot lysis	1	
c	Increased (i) → give fresh frozen plasma (FFP)	1	*Normal ranges for the parameters derived from point-of-care coagulation testing vary between devices.*
	Decreased (ii) → give cryoprecipitate/fibrinogen	1	
	Decreased (iii) → give platelet transfusion	1	
	Decreased (iv) → give tranexamic acid	1	
d	• Whole blood added to cup(s) at 37°C • Pin suspended in cup • Cup rotates • As blood clots, rotational movement of cup is transmitted to the pin • Torsion wire connected to pin • Electrical transducer converts torsion on the pin into a graph	Any 5	*The ROTEM® uses a variation of this technology:* • *A pin is immersed into the blood, the cuvette is stationary* • *Increasing impedance is detected by an optical system*
e	360 μL (TEG®) or 300 μL (ROTEM®)	1	

Suggested reading

A. Srivastava, A. Kelleher. Point-of-care coagulation testing. *Cont Edu Anaesth Crit Care Pain* 2013; **13**: 12–6.

Paper 10 Answers

Question 1 Seizure

Q	Marking guidance	Mark	Comments
a	• Epilepsy: either known history or first fit • Metabolic: hypoglycaemia, hyponatraemia (maximum 1 mark for metabolic causes) • Intracranial pathology: haemorrhage, tumour, infection (meningitis, encephalitis, HIV) (maximum 2 marks for intracranial causes) • Poisoning Not acceptable: febrile convulsion (typically age 6 months to 5 years)	Any 4	*Two seizures are required before epilepsy can be diagnosed.*
b	• Focal seizure (also known as partial seizure) • Absence seizure (also known as petit mal) • Atonic seizure (also known as drop attack) • Clonic seizure • Tonic seizure • Myoclonic seizure	Any 3	*The patient may retain awareness (simple partial seizure) or lose awareness (complex partial seizure).*
c	• ABC assessment • Confirm clinically that this is a seizure • Apply oxygen • Establish IV access • Blood glucose • Venous blood gas for Na$^+$	Any 3	

(cont.)

Q	Marking guidance	Mark	Comments
d	<u>5 min:</u>		Must have drug and per kg dose to gain each mark.
	• Midazolam 0.5 mg/kg buccal	1	
	• Lorazepam 0.1 mg/kg IV	1	
	<u>15 min:</u>		
	Lorazepam 0.1 mg/kg IV	1	
	<u>25 min:</u>		
	• Phenytoin 20 mg/kg IV infusion over 20 min	1	
	• Phenobarbital 20 mg/kg IV over 5 min	1	
	<u>45 min:</u>		
	Thiopentone 4 mg/kg IV (accept 3–6 mg/kg)	1	
e	• 6.0 mm uncuffed ETT • 5.5 mm cuffed ETT	Any 1	*Formula is (age/4)+4 for uncuffed ETTs, with 0.5 mm subtracted for cuffed ETTs.*
f	Size CD = 460 L (accept 400–600 L) Size E = 680 L (accept 600–800 L) Size F = 1360 L (accept 1200–1500 L)	3	

Suggested reading

National Institute for Health and Care Excellence. Clinical guideline 137, Appendix F: Protocols for treating convulsive status epilepticus in adults and children, 2011. www.nice.org.uk/guidance/cg137/chapter/Appendix-F-Protocols-for-treating-convulsive-status-epilepticus-in-adults-and-children-adults-published-in-2004-and-children-published-in-2011#guidelines-for-treating-convulsive-status-epilepticus-in-children-published-in-2011. (Accessed 28 October 2018).

A. R. Barakat, S. Mallory. Anaesthesia and childhood epilepsy. *Cont Edu Anaesth Crit Care Pain* 2011; **11**(3): 93–8.

Question 2 Off-Pump Cardiac Bypass

Q	Marking guidance	Mark	Comments
a	• Aortic disease precluding bypass • Renal disease • Ventricular dysfunction • Diabetes • Advanced age • Chronic lung disease • Previous cerebrovascular accident (CVA)	Any 4	*In off-pump procedures:* • *aortic cannulation is not required, which reduces the risk of aortic dissection or embolisation.* • *an aortic cross-clamp is not required, which reduces the risk of plaque embolism and subsequent CVA.* *Patients who are at higher risk of complications from conventional cardiopulmonary bypass may benefit from off-pump surgery.*
b	250–300 s	1	*A typical dose of heparin to achieve this degree of anticoagulation is 1–2 mg/kg (100–200 U/kg).*
c	• Need upward blood flow into vertically positioned ventricle	1	*A greater filling pressure is required to maintain ventricular filling.*
	• Vertical position distorts mitral and tricuspid annuli	1	*Distortion of annuli can result in significant valvular regurgitation.*
d	• Trendelenburg position • Fluid administration • Commencement of noradrenaline • Atrial pacing to a rate of 60 beats/min	Any 3	*Target mean arterial pressure should be > 70 mmHg.*

(cont.)

Q	Marking guidance	Mark	Comments
e	**Esmolol:** • Receptor activity: β_1-adrenoreceptor antagonist • Metabolism: red cell esterases • Affected phase: phase 4	3	*Esmolol is highly cardio-selective, has rapid onset and offset and has a metabolism independent of liver or renal function. The gradient of phase 4 of the pacemaker potential is reduced, thus decreasing heart rate.*
	Verapamil: • Receptor activity: competitive calcium channel blocker • Metabolism: hepatic metabolism • Affected phase: phase 0	3	*Verapamil is a specific antagonist of the L-type Ca^{2+} channel, with a particular affinity for those at the SA and AV nodes.*
f	• Requires fewer staff (no perfusionist) • Reduced transfusion costs • Reduced length of stay • Reduced number of ventilated days • Reduced equipment requirements (no bypass circuit)	Any 4	

Suggested reading

D. Hett. Anaesthesia for off-pump coronary artery surgery. *Cont Edu Anaesth Crit Care Pain* 2006; **6**(2): 60–2.

Question 3 Acute Respiratory Distress Syndrome (ARDS)

Q	Marking guidance	Mark	Comments
a	• Timing: within 1 week of the start of symptoms • Chest imaging: bilateral opacities • Not explained entirely by fluid overload • P_aO_2/F_iO_2 ratio < 39.9 (accept a ratio < 300 when using mmHg) (minimum PEEP of 5 cmH$_2$O)	1 1 1 1	*Causes of ARDS may be classified as follows:* • *Direct causes: pneumonia, aspiration, lung contusion, fat embolism, drowning, inhalational injury, reperfusion injury.* • *Indirect causes: sepsis, multiple trauma, massive transfusion, pancreatitis, cardiopulmonary bypass.*
b	• Ventilation using 6–8 mL/kg tidal volume • Permissive hypercapnia • High positive end-expiratory pressure (PEEP) • Plateau pressure < 30 cmH$_2$O • Recruitment manoeuvres • Avoid hyperoxia	Any 4	*A pH > 7.20 is commonly accepted; the actual P_aCO_2 is of lesser importance.*
c	• Improved $\dot{V}/\dot{Q}$ ratio • Increase in functional residual capacity • Recruitment of atelectatic lung	3	*Displacement of the heart which compresses surrounding lung tissue also helps improve $\dot{V}/\dot{Q}$ matching.*
d	• P_aO_2/F_iO_2 on 100% O_2 • PEEP (cmH$_2$O) • Compliance (mL/cmH$_2$O) • Chest X-ray quadrants infiltrated	4	*Each component scored from 0 to 4. A Murray score ≥ 3 represents severe respiratory failure appropriate for referral for extracorporeal membrane oxygenation (ECMO).*

(cont.)

Q	Marking guidance	Mark	Comments
e	• High peak inspiratory pressures > 30 cmH$_2$O for more than 7 days • High F_iO_2 ventilation (>0.8) for more than 7 days • Intracranial bleed • Any other contraindication to heparinisation	4	*To be eligible, patients must have a reversible cause of respiratory failure and should not have a life-limiting comorbidity aside from the acute disease process.*
f	Veno-venous circuit	1	

Suggested reading

V. McCormack, S. Tolhurst-Cleaver. Acute respiratory distress syndrome. *BJA Education* 2017; **17**(5): 161–5.

G. Martinez, A. Vuylsteke. Extracorporeal membrane oxygenation in adults. *Cont Edu Anaesth Crit Care Pain* 2012: **12**(2): 57–61.

Question 4 Strabismus Surgery

Q	Marking guidance	Mark	Comments
a	• Down's syndrome • Edward's syndrome • Cri du chat • Goldenhar • Treacher–Collins • Smith–Lemli–Opitz • Crouzon • Apert • Pfeiffer	Any 2	
b	• Soft • Early systolic • Varies with position • No abnormal signs/symptoms (e.g. failure to thrive, syncope, cyanosis)	Any 3	*A murmur should be investigated prior to surgery in the following situations:* • *<1 year old* • *Pathological murmurs (all diastolic, pansystolic, late systolic, loud or continuous murmurs)* • *Any abnormal symptoms or signs* • *Abnormal ECG or chest X-ray.*
c	Paracetamol: 15 mg/kg (accept 20 mg/kg) Ibuprofen: 5 mg/kg Glycopyrrolate: 4–8 µg/kg Ondansetron: 0.1–0.15 mg/kg Dexamethasone: 0.15 mg/kg	5	*Strabismus surgery can cause severe pain. A common analgesic regimen is topical local anaesthetic, opioid analgesia, e.g. fentanyl, paracetamol and ibuprofen; multimodal analgesia should be continued into the post-operative period. The use of opioids increases the risk of post-operative nausea and vomiting (PONV), and antiemetics are essential.*

(cont.)

Q	Marking guidance	Mark	Comments
d	Reflex: oculocardiac Afferent: ophthalmic division (V$_1$) of trigeminal nerve Efferent: vagus nerve	1 1 1	*The relay for the oculocardiac reflex is via the sensory nucleus in the fourth ventricle.* *Children with a positive oculocardiac reflex are more likely to develop PONV than those with no measurable reflex. It has been postulated that preventing the oculocardiac reflex may reduce the incidence of PONV.*
e	<u>Patient-related factors:</u> • Term baby < 1 month in age • Preterm or ex-preterm baby < 60 weeks post-conception age • Poorly controlled systemic disease • Inborn errors of metabolism (including diabetes mellitus) • Complex cardiac disease or cardiac disease requiring investigation • Sickle cell disease (not trait) • Active infection (especially of respiratory tract) <u>Social factors:</u> • Parent unable to care for the child at home post-operatively • Poor housing conditions • No telephone • Excessive journey time from home to the hospital (>1 hour) • Inadequate post-operative transport arrangement	Any 4 Any 3	*Anaesthetic/operative factors that preclude paediatric day-case surgery include:* • *Inexperienced surgeon or anaesthetist* • *Prolonged procedure* • *Opening of a body cavity* • *High risk of perioperative haemorrhage/fluid loss* • *Post-operative pain unlikely to be relieved by oral analgesics* • *Difficult airway (including obstructive sleep apnoea)* • *Malignant hyperpyrexia susceptibility* • *Sibling of a victim of sudden infant death syndrome*

Suggested reading

N. Shetty, D. Sethi. Paediatric anaesthesia for day surgery. World Federation of Societies of Anaesthesiologists' Anaesthesia Tutorial of the Week 203, 2010. www.aagbi.org/sites/def ault/files/203-Anaesthesia-for-paediatric-day-surgery.pdf. (Accessed 2 October 2018).

G. Stuart. Anaesthesia for paediatric eye surgery. World Federation of Societies of Anaesthesiologists' Anaesthesia Tutorial of the Week 144, 2009. www.aagbi.org/sites/def ault/files/144-anaesthesia-for-paediatric-eye-surgery.pdf. (Accessed 2 October 2018).

Question 5 Post-partum Cardiomyopathy

Q	Marking guidance	Mark	Comments
a	• Development of heart failure within the last month of pregnancy or up to 5 months following delivery	1	*PPCM closely resembles dilated cardiomyopathy.*
	• Absence of another identifiable cause of heart failure	1	
	• Left ventricular systolic dysfunction on echocardiogram/ejection fraction < 45%	1	
b	• Left axis deviation • T-wave inversion (lateral leads/III) • Presence of Q waves (III/aVF) • Atrial/ventricular ectopics • Sinus tachycardia	Any 3	*The heart is physiologically dilated and displaced in both cephalad and lateral directions.* *Increasing circulating vasopressors and diaphragmatic changes may play a role.*
c	• Hypertensive disorders • Maternal age > 30 years • Multiparity • Multiple pregnancy • Obesity • Cocaine use • Afro-Caribbean descent	Any 5	
d	• Invasive arterial monitoring • Maintain preload/left lateral tilt to avoid aortocaval compression • Avoid tachycardia • Avoid increases in afterload • Maintain sinus rhythm • Maintain contractility • Avoid hypotension/carefully titrated spinal block • Avoid fluid overload/cautious intravenous infusion/furosemide on delivery	Any 5	*Vaginal delivery is favoured with low dose epidural analgesia.* *Effective analgesia will help prevent tachycardia.* *Assisted second stage can reduce cardiovascular instability.*

(cont.)

Q	Marking guidance	Mark	Comments
e	Oxytocin: • Decrease in systemic vascular resistance/compensatory tachycardia • Coronary vasoconstriction Ergometrine: • Coronary vasoconstriction • Pulmonary vasoconstriction • Systemic vasoconstriction		*Oxytocin must be slowly titrated.* *Ergometrine should be avoided in patients with PPCM.*

Suggested reading

C. Burt, J. Durbridge. Management of cardiac disease in pregnancy. *Cont Edu Anaesth Crit Care Pain* 2009; **9**(2): 44–7.

V. Regitz-Zagrosek, J. W. Roos-Hesselink, J. Bauersachs, et al. 2018 ESC Guidelines for the management of cardiovascular diseases during pregnancy. *Eur Heart J* 2018; **39**(34): 3165–241.

Question 6 Spinal Cord Stimulator

Q	Marking guidance	Mark	Comments
a	• Failed back surgery syndrome • Complex regional pain syndrome • Neuropathic pain secondary to peripheral nerve damage • Ischaemic pain associated with peripheral vascular disease Not acceptable: chronic back pain	Any 2	*These are the four indications recommended by the National Institute for Health and Care Excellence (Technology appraisal guidance TA159).*
b	• Psychological unsuitability: personality disorder, significant depression/anxiety • Uncontrolled bleeding/anticoagulation • Systemic or severe sepsis • Implanted cardiac devices: demand pacemaker or defibrillator • Immunosuppression	Any 2	
c	• Stimulator leads: 4–8 electrodes, either paddles (surgically placed) or catheters (percutaneously placed) • Pulse generator: external (for spinal cord stimulator trial) or implanted	1 1	*The pulse generator is usually implanted subcutaneously in the anterior abdominal wall, lateral chest wall, gluteal or infraclavicular areas.*
d	• Avoid unipolar diathermy if possible • If not possible, place neutral plate so that SCS components are outside the electrical field of diathermy • Risk of damaging/causing infection of leads with neuraxial blockade • Care with patient positioning/padding of SCS pulse generator	Any 2	*There is no need to give patients antibiotic prophylaxis specifically due to the presence of an SCS.*

Q	Marking guidance	Mark	Comments
e	• Rectus sheath block/catheters • Bilateral transverse abdominis plane block/catheters • Wound catheters • Surgical infiltration of the wound • Lignocaine infusion Not acceptable: neuraxial techniques, due to presence of SCS	Any 4	*Lignocaine infusions are increasingly commonly used for intra-operative analgesia. An ongoing lignocaine infusion mandates a bed in a higher care area.*
f	• Clonidine 1 μg/kg intravenous • Ketamine 0.2–0.75 mg/kg intravenous • Lignocaine 1.5 mg/kg intravenous	3	
g	• Agitation/restlessness • Anxiety • Muscle aches • Insomnia • Rhinorrhoea/tears • Sweating • Yawning • Tachycardia/tachypnoea	Any 3	*Symptoms such as goose bumps, dilated pupils and abdominal cramps are later symptoms.*
h	• Oral oxycodone:oral morphine ratio is 1: 2	1	
	• Oral morphine:intravenous morphine ratio is 3:1	1	*The different opioid equivalence of oral and intravenous morphine is due to first-pass metabolism.*

Suggested reading

G. K. Simpson, M. Jackson. Perioperative management of opioid-tolerant patients. *BJA Education* 2017; **17**(4): 124–8.

S. Ramaswamy, J. A. Wilson, L. Colvin. Non-opioid-based adjunct analgesia in perioperative care. *Cont Edu Anaesth Crit Care Pain* 2013; **13**(5): 152–7.

J. H. Raphael, H. S. Mutagi, S. Kapur. Spinal cord stimulation and its anaesthetic implications. *Cont Edu Anaesth Crit Care Pain* 2009; **9**(3): 78–81.

Question 7 Enhanced Recovery

Q	Marking guidance	Mark	Comments
a	• Interleukin 1 (IL-1) • Interleukin 6 (IL-6) • Tumour necrosis factor alpha (TNF-α)	Any 2	*Cytokines contribute to the haematological consequences of the surgical stress response, including* • *hypercoagulability* • *fibrinolysis.*
b	Cortisol: • Increased protein breakdown • Promotes gluconeogenesis • Increased lipolysis • Peripheral insulin resistance/ hyperglycaemia • Anti-inflammatory activity/ immunomodulatory effect Growth hormone: • Increased protein synthesis • Reduced proteolysis • Promotes lipolysis • Anti-insulin effect • Glycogenolysis	Any 2 Any 2	*Other hormones implicated in the surgical stress response include the following:* • *Antidiuretic hormone (increased secretion)* • *Insulin (reduced secretion)* • *Adrenocorticotrophic hormone (increased secretion)* • *β-endorphin (increased secretion)* • *Prolactin (increased secretion).* *The other major contributor in the surgical stress response is the activation of the sympathetic nervous system.*

(cont.)

Q	Marking guidance	Mark	Comments
c	Option 1: Oral iron therapy	1	*Anaemia may be corrected*
	Advantages:	Any 1	*by allogenic transfusion, but*
	• Ease of administration		*it is now established that*
	• Low cost		*transfusion itself is*
	Disadvantages:	Any 1	*associated with increased*
	• Poor tolerance/gastrointestinal side effects		*perioperative morbidity and mortality.*
	• Poor bioavailability		*Treatment of pre-operative*
	• Limited time for effect		*anaemia should be directed*
	Option 2: Intravenous iron therapy	1	*at correcting the underlying*
	Advantages:	Any 1	*cause. Correcting anaemia*
	• More effective rise in haemoglobin		*before surgery reduces perioperative transfusion*
	• Adequate time frame for effect		*rates, post-operative*
	Disadvantages:	Any 1	*infective and ischaemic*
	• Requires hospital admission		*complications and length of*
	• Risk of anaphylaxis		*hospital stay. It also conserves blood stocks and is associated with cost savings.*
d	• Administration of a 250 mL crystalloid fluid bolus	1	
	• Observation of changes in stroke volume over subsequent 10 min	1	
	• An increase in stroke volume of < 10% means a further bolus of IV fluid is not indicated. An increase in stroke volume of > 10% means a further fluid bolus should be administered	1	
e	• Use of short-acting anaesthetic agents	Any 2	*There is little evidence to favour one anaesthetic technique over another, but the general principles of enhanced recovery support the use of agents that have minimal post-operative hang-over and effects on gastrointestinal motility.*

(cont.)

Q	Marking guidance	Mark	Comments
	• Multi-modal analgesia/ avoidance of long-acting opioids		
	• Temperature homeostasis		
	• Risk stratification/prophylaxis against post-operative nausea and vomiting		*Total intravenous anaesthesia can be used and may play an increasing role in cancer surgery in the future.*
	• Consideration of regional anaesthesia		*Neuraxial blockade offers advantages over other regional techniques, such as* • *reduction in the duration of ileus* • *reduced blood loss* • *reduction in post-operative pulmonary complications, including pulmonary embolism* • *modification of the stress response.* *However, potential disadvantages include* • *complications associated with their insertion* • *reduced mobilisation* • *excessive fluid administration to combat hypotension.*
f	• Multi-modal analgesia/ avoidance of excessive intravenous opiates • Early discontinuation of intravenous fluids/early enteral intake • Early removal of drains/ catheters	Any 3	*Another vital part of enhanced recovery is audit to review compliance with the pathway.*

(cont.)

Q	Marking guidance	Mark	Comments
	• Early mobilisation • Multi-disciplinary approach to post-operative care • Telephone follow-up on discharge		

Suggested reading

C. Matthews. Enhanced recovery after surgery (ERAS). World Federation of Societies of Anaesthesiologists' Anaesthesia Tutorial of the Week 204, 2010. www.aagbi.org/sites/default/files/204-Enhanced-recovery-after-surgery-ERAS.pdf. (Accessed 3 October 2018).

L. J. S. Kelliher, C. N. Jones, W. J. Fawcett. Enhanced recovery for gastrointestinal surgery. *Cont Edu Anaesth Crit Care Pain* 2015; 15(6): 305–10.

G. A. Hans, N. Jones. Preoperative anaemia. *Cont Edu Anaesth Crit Care Pain* 2013; 13(3): 71–4.

Question 8   Blood Transfusion

Q	Marking guidance	Mark	Comments
a	<u>Major haemorrhage</u> • Loss of total blood volume within 24 hours • Loss of 50% blood volume in < 3 hours • Bleeding in excess of 150 mL/min • Bleeding leading to a systolic blood pressure of < 90 mmHg and pulse of > 110 beats/min	Any 1	*There is no one accepted definition for either major haemorrhage or massive transfusion.*
	<u>Massive transfusion</u> • Transfusion of ≥10 red blood cell (RBC) units within 24 hours • Transfusion of >4 RBC units within 1 hour, with anticipation of continued need for blood product support • Replacement of > 50% of the total blood volume by blood products within 3 hours	Any 1	
b	<u>Component:</u> metabolic acidosis	1	*Early trauma-induced coagulopathy (ETIC) is associated with systemic anticoagulation and hyperfibrinolysis.*
	<u>Consequence:</u>	Any 1	
	• pH affects activity of factors V, VIIa and X • Acidosis inhibits thrombin		*Tissue injury from trauma releases local and systemic tissue factor which activates coagulation pathways.*
	<u>Component:</u> hypothermia	1	
	<u>Consequence:</u>	Any 1	*The initiation results in massive consumptive coagulopathy leading to a consumptive disseminated*
	• Decreases platelet activation • Increases platelet sequestration in liver and spleen • Reduces functions of factors XI and XII • Inhibits fibrinolysis		

Q	Marking guidance	Mark	Comments
	<u>Component</u>: acute coagulopathy	1	*intravascular coagulation-like syndrome, most commonly seen in patients with severe head injury or extensive muscle damage.*
	<u>Consequence</u>: • Systemic anticoagulation • Consumption of coagulation factors • Hyperfibrinolysis	Any 1	
c	• RBCs: haemoglobin >80 g/L (accept 70–90 g/L)	1	
	• Fresh frozen plasma: international normalised ratio (INR) < 1.5/prothrombin time < 15 s.	1	
	• Cryoprecipitate: fibrinogen > 1.5 g/L	1	*Fibrinogen target is > 2 g/L in obstetric haemorrhage*
	• Platelets: platelet count > 75 ×10^9/L	1	
d	<u>Transfusion reactions</u>: • Allergic reaction (accept urticaria/anaphylaxis) • Haemolytic transfusion reaction • Febrile non-haemolytic transfusion reaction	Any 2	*Other complications include the following:* • *Infection* • *Transfusion-associated circulatory overload (TACO) (infants and patients with pre-existing cardiac disease are at increased risk)* • *Air embolism: rare and potentially fatal complication of rapid infusor use.*
	<u>Immunological reactions</u>: • Transfusion-related acute lung injury (TRALI) • Transfusion-related immunomodulation (TRIM) • Transfusion-associated graft vs host disease (Ta-GVHD) • Post-transfusion purpura (PTP)	Any 2	
	<u>Metabolic complications</u>: • Hypocalcaemia	Any 2	*Hypocalcaemia due to citrate overload.*
	• Hypomagnesaemia • Hyperkalaemia		*Hyperkalaemia is due to haemolysis of RBCs during storage, irradiation or both.*
	• Hypokalaemia		

(cont.)

Q	Marking guidance	Mark	Comments
			Hypokalaemia may occur because of K⁺ re-entry into transfused RBCs.
	• Metabolic alkalosis		*Metabolic alkalosis may occur because of citrate overload.*
	• Metabolic acidosis		*Metabolic acidosis occurs because of hypoperfusion, liver dysfunction and citrate overload.*
	• Hypothermia		*Hypothermia occurs through conduction: infusion of cold blood products. A blood warmer should always be used.*
e	<u>Pharmacodynamic effect:</u> Competitive inhibitor of conversion of plasminogen to active plasmin	1	
	<u>Dose:</u> 1 g intravenous bolus, followed by infusion of a further 1 g over 8 hours	1	Both bolus and infusion doses needed for 1 mark.

Suggested reading

A. Klein, P. Arnold, R. M. Bingham, et al. AAGBI guidelines: the use of blood components and their alternatives. *Anaesthesia* 2016; **71**(7): 829–42.

H. P. Pham, B. H. Shaz. Update on massive transfusion. *Br J Anaes* 2013; **111**(1): 71–82.

T. C. Nicholson, R. Berry. Pre-hospital trauma care and aero-medical transfer: a military perspective. *Cont Edu Anaesth Crit Care Pain* 2012; **12**(4): 186–9.

Question 9   Physical Injuries

Q	Marking guidance	Mark	Comments
a	Causes of corneal abrasion: • Direct trauma • Exposure keratopathy • Chemical injury Physical prevention measures: • Taping of the eyelid • Instillation of ointment • Bio-occlusive dressings • Use of non-toxic antiseptic	 1 1 1 Any 3	Clinical features of corneal abrasions are pain, gritty sensation, redness, tearing and photophobia. The diagnosis may be confirmed with fluorescein staining and slit lamp examination. Treatment includes lubricants and topical antibiotics. Occasionally patching of the eye or bandage lens is required.
b	• Weakness of dorsiflexion • Foot drop • Weakness of eversion • Weakness of extensor hallucis longus • Paraesthesia over the dorsal aspect of the foot/lower lateral part of the leg	Any 3	Common peroneal nerve palsy is classically described following surgery in the lithotomy position and is due to pressure on the common peroneal nerve as it passes in close proximity to the head of the fibula.
c	• Ulnar nerve injury • Brachial plexus injury	1 1	
d	• Pre-operative dental review • Use laryngeal mask airway (LMA) over an endotracheal tube • Use regional anaesthesia/neuraxial blockade • Blind nasal intubation • Bite block • Deep extubation • Senior operator	Any 4	If a tooth is avulsed, relocate it as soon as possible and apply pressure or a splint. Apologise and explain to patient, offer analgesia and refer to a dentist.

(cont.)

Q	Marking guidance	Mark	Comments
e	• Larger diameter endotracheal tubes • Poor endotracheal insertion technique (accept trauma)/ difficult intubation • High endotracheal cuff pressures • Duration of anaesthesia • Use of nasogastric tubes • Use of non-humidified breathing systems	Any 5	*Around 20% of patients report a sore throat following LMA insertion and 40% of patients after endotracheal intubation. Symptoms persisting over 48 hours should be investigated.*

Suggested reading

D. W. Hewson, J. G. Hardman. Physical injuries during anaesthesia. *BJA Educ* 2018; **18**(10): 310–6.

Question 10 Fractured Neck of Femur

Q	Marking guidance	Mark	Comments
a	Less than 36–48 hours	1	*Surgery should be performed within 48 hours of hospital admission after hip fracture.* *A target of 36 hours was introduced in England and Wales in April 2010.*
b	• Full blood count • Urea and electrolytes • Coagulation screen/ international normalised ratio (INR) • Group and save/hold • Electrocardiogram (ECG)	Any 4	*A coagulation screen is only required where clinically indicated (e.g. patient taking oral anticoagulants). Chest X-ray is only indicated in specific circumstances, e.g. newly diagnosed cardiac failure or suspected pneumonia.*
c	• Breathless at rest/on minimal exertion • A history of angina on exertion • Unexplained syncope • A slow rising pulse • Absent second heart sound	Any 2	*Echocardiography is also indicated if there is evidence of left ventricular hypertrophy on ECG without a history of hypertension.*
d	• Haemoglobin concentration < 80 g/L • Plasma sodium < 120 mmol/L or > 150 mmol/L • Plasma potassium < 2.8 mmol/L or > 6.0 mmol/L • Uncontrolled diabetes • Uncontrolled or acute onset left ventricular failure • Chest infection with sepsis • Reversible coagulopathy • Correctable cardiac arrhythmia with a ventricular rate > 120 beats/min	Any 3	*The AAGBI gives the following as unacceptable reasons to delay surgery:* • *Lack of facilities or theatre space* • *Awaiting echocardiography* • *Unavailable surgical expertise* • *Minor electrolyte abnormalities*

(cont.)

Q	Marking guidance	Mark	Comments
e	• Device: cardiac output monitor (accept oesophageal Doppler, LiDCO, etc.) • Reason: to provide goal-directed fluid therapy/improve haemodynamic performance • Device: depth of anaesthesia monitor (accept bispectral index, E-entropy, etc.) • Reason: avoid potential cardiovascular depression from excessive anaesthesia • Device: central venous pressure monitoring • Reason: guide intra-operative fluid therapy (do not accept for drug delivery) • Device: cerebral oxygen saturation monitoring • Reason: reduce post-operative cognitive dysfunction through early recognition and management of reduced intra-operative cerebral oxygen saturations	4	1 mark for each correct device (maximum 2 marks). 1 mark for each correct corresponding reason (maximum 2 marks).
f	• Damage to abdominal viscera • Retroperitoneal haematoma • Psoas abscess • Epidural spread • Intrathecal injection	Any 3	*Unlike a psoas compartment block, a femoral nerve/fascia iliaca block does not reliably block the obturator nerve. However, a femoral nerve/fascia iliaca block is more amenable to ultrasound-guided placement and still significantly reduces post-operative analgesic requirements.*

Q	Marking guidance	Mark	Comments
g	6–24 hours	1	*Some centres re-instigate warfarin therapy on the day of surgery.*
h	• Utilising a lower dose of intrathecal bupivacaine • Using intrathecal fentanyl to facilitate a reduced dose of intrathecal bupivacaine • Using hyperbaric bupivacaine with the patient positioned laterally (fractured hip lowermost)	Any 2	

Suggested reading

Association of Anaesthetists of Great Britain and Ireland. Management of proximal femoral fractures. *Anaesthesia* 2012; 67(1): 85–98.

R. Cheung. Neck of femur fracture; perioperative management. World Federation of Societies of Anaesthesiologists' Anaesthesia Tutorial of the Week 296, 2013. www.aagbi.org/sites/default/files/296%20Neck%20of%20Femur%20Fractu re;%20Peri-operative%20Management[1].pdf. (Accessed 2 October 2018).

Question 11   Oxygen and Carbon Dioxide Transport

Q	Marking guidance	Mark	Comments
a	• Four polypeptide chains/two alpha and two beta chains • Four haem moieties/porphyrin rings with iron atoms • Iron in ferrous state • Chains bound together by hydrogen bonds	Any 3	*In adults 95% of haemoglobin (Hb) exists in the form of HbA1 containing two alpha and two beta chains. Foetal Hb consists of two alpha and two gamma chains.*
b	Oxygen (O_2) binding: • O_2 forms a reversible bond to ferrous iron in Hb • There are four O_2 binding sites/four O_2 molecules bind • Each ferrous iron binds a molecule of O_2/each Hb molecule binds four O_2 molecules Cooperative binding: Binding of an O_2 molecule to Hb increases Hb's affinity for O_2, facilitating the uptake of additional O_2 molecules	Any 2 1	*Cooperative binding is explained by allosteric modulation: when O_2 binds to Hb, the two beta chains move closer together and the haem moieties adopt a 'relaxed' state which has an increased affinity for O_2. When O_2 dissociates from Hb the 'taut' state is favoured, reducing Hb's affinity for O_2.*
c	• Increased pH/alkalosis • Reduced P_aCO_2 • Reduced 2,3-diphosphoglycerate • Reduced temperature • Carboxyhaemoglobin • Methaemoglobinaemia Not acceptable: foetal Hb, as the question asks specifically about adult Hb	Any 4	*This question is looking for factors that shift the adult oxyhaemoglobin dissociation curve to the left.*

Q	Marking guidance	Mark	Comments
d	• Hypoxaemic hypoxia: due to reduced P_aO_2	1	*Hypoxaemic hypoxia has a number of causes, e.g.* • *inadvertent low inspired O_2* • *hypoventilation* • *$\dot{V}/\dot{Q}$ mismatch* • *diffusion impairment.*
	• Anaemic hypoxia: P_aO_2 is normal, but oxygen carrying capacity is reduced	1	*Anaemic hypoxia may be due to anaemia or carbon monoxide poisoning.*
	• Stagnant hypoxia: normal arterial oxygen content, circulatory failure leading to inadequate oxygen delivery	1	*Stagnant hypoxia may be seen in cardiogenic shock.*
	• Histotoxic/cytotoxic hypoxia: normal arterial oxygen content and delivery to tissues, but an inability of tissues to utilise O_2 at a cellular level	1	*Cyanide inhibits cytochrome c oxidase in the mitochondrial electron transport chain, resulting in histotoxic hypoxia.*
e	• Dissolved • Carbamino compounds, or bound to haemoglobin • As bicarbonate or carbonic acid	1 1 1	*CO_2 diffuses into red blood cell, combines with water to form carbonic acid (catalysed by carbonic anhydrase) which dissociates to form bicarbonate. Bicarbonate diffuses out of red blood cells and is carried in the plasma.*
f	Carbonic anhydrase	1	

(cont.)

Q	Marking guidance	Mark	Comments
g	<u>Haldane effect:</u> Increased ability of deoxygenated haemoglobin to carry carbon dioxide	1	*The double Haldane effect describes how maternal uptake of CO_2 increases whilst foetal CO_2 affinity decreases, enhancing the transfer of CO_2 from foetal to maternal circulations.*
	<u>Relevance:</u> • In the tissues, increases affinity for carbon dioxide • In the lungs, decreased affinity facilitates removal of carbon dioxide	Any 1	

Suggested reading

J.-O. C. Dunn, M. P. Grocott. Physiology of oxygen transport. *BJA Educ* 2016; **16**(10): 341–8.

G. J. Arthurs, M. Sudhakar. Carbon dioxide transport. *Cont Edu Anaesth Crit Care Pain* 2005; **5**(6): 207–10.

Question 12 Laser

Q	Marking guidance	Mark	Comments
a	Light Amplification by Stimulated Emission of Radiation	1	*Albert Einstein published the theoretical basis for laser in 1917, but it was only in 1960 that the first functioning laser was constructed.*
b	Monochromatic	1	*Monochromatic: consisting of a single wavelength or colour.*
	Coherent	1	*Coherent: photons are in phase.*
	Collimated	1	*Collimated: photons are almost in parallel (aligned), with little divergence from the point of origin.*
c	Spontaneous emission = photon is released from an electron that has spontaneously returned to ground state from a higher energy state	1	
	Stimulated emission = a photon collides with an electron in a higher energy orbit, causing a photon to be released as the electron decays back to ground state	1	*Stimulated emission is provoked in a lasing medium through the use of reflective mirrors which reflect photons back into the lasing medium, encouraging further collision. The photons are released in phase and in the same direction as the stimulating photon.*
	Population inversion: where more electrons exist in higher excited states than in lower unexcited states	1	*Population inversion is achieved by continuous input from the energy pump (continuous wave laser) or by intermittent pumping (pulsed wave laser).*

(cont.)

Q	Marking guidance	Mark	Comments
d	i) Carbon dioxide (CO_2)	1	*A CO_2 laser utilises a photo-thermal effect, rapidly heating tissues. Depending on the exposure time, tissue vapourisation (ablation), coagulation or both may occur.*
	ii) Accept lithotripsy, endoscopic sinus surgery or tissue ablation	1	*Holmium:YAG laser utilises a photo-mechanical effect. It causes an extremely intense but brief pulse of laser. This results in explosive expansion of the tissue or water within the renal calculi, causing photoacoustic disruption.*
	iii) Accept: excimer or argon fluoride	1	*These lasers break down covalent bonds in protein molecules (photodissociation), resulting in non-thermal ablation.*
e	• Saline filled cuff • Methylene blue/dye-filled cuff • Twin distal cuffs • PVC tube wrapped with self-adhesive, non-reflective metal tape	Any 2	*Cuffs of endotracheal tubes are vulnerable to rupture by laser beams. If a cuff inflated with air is ruptured, it allows a massive leak of anaesthetic gases and provides a richer environment for ignition.*

Q	Marking guidance	Mark	Comments
f	• Protective goggles (glasses/spectacles not acceptable, as they do not give reliable peripheral visual field protection)	Any 3	*The protective eyewear must correspond to the wavelength of laser light being used.*
	• Divergent laser beam		*To reduce the risk of focussed laser light striking the retina.*
	• Matt-black surgical instruments		*To minimise reflection from the main laser beam.*
	• Appropriately trained designated laser safety officer		
	• 'Laser in use' signage/locked theatre doors/theatre windows covered		*To prevent accidental injury to passers-by.*
	• Non-water based fire extinguisher available		
g	• Declare incident/call for help	Any 5	*Further (non-immediate) management may include:*
	• Discontinue use of laser		
	• Stop ventilation/discontinue oxygen source		*• Tracheostomy*
	• Remove the burnt endotracheal tube		*• Steroid therapy to treat inflammation*
	• Douse the operative site with water		*• Antibiotic therapy*
	• Reinstate ventilation with bag–mask ventilation or re-intubation using room air		*• Transfer to critical care for ventilatory support if concerned about upper airway swelling or lung injury.*
	• Perform bronchoscopy to determine degree of thermal injury		

Suggested reading

E. Simpson. The basic principles of laser technology, uses and safety measures in anaesthesia. World Federation of Societies of Anaesthesiologists' Anaesthesia Tutorial of the Week 255, 2012. www.aagbi.org/sites/default/files/255%20Basic%20Principles%20of%20Laser%20Technology.pdf. (Accessed 27 September 2018).

Index

Answers are denoted by page numbers in **bold**

abdominal aortic aneurysm
(AAA), 13, **146–147**
abdominal compression, 15
abnormal placental
adherence, 43
accidental awareness under
general anaesthesia, 32,
192–193
psychological harm, **192**
acidosis, 40, **210**
acoustic artefacts, 97, **345**
acoustic neuroma, 62, **263–264**
acromegaly, **235**
activated charcoal, 81, **307**
activated clotting time (ACT),
90, 112
acute asthma, 64–65, **268–269**
life-threatening, 64, **268**
ventilator settings, 65, **269**
acute kidney injury (AKI), 13
acute myeloid leukaemia, **186**
acute respiratory distress
syndrome (ARDS),
113, **383**
addiction, **372**
adrenalectomy, 33
adrenaline, **196**
afterload, 108, **374**
airway burns, 48–49, **233–234**
airway fire, 122, **409**
alcohol abuse, 94
alfentanil, 28, 95, **338**
allogenic transfusion, 11
amitriptyline, 12, **142**
amniotic fluid embolism, 30,
188–189
incidence and death
from, **188**
amputation, phantom limb
pain and, 67, 68, **274**
anaemia
pre-operative, 11, **140–141**,
393
renal failure and, **280**
anaesthesia. *See also* regional
anaesthesia, general
anaesthesia

spinal, 54, 96, 104, 115, **245**
total intravenous, 23–24, 47,
173–174
analgesia
caudal, 6, 7, **129–130**
hip fracture, 80, **305**
labour and, 103–104,
363–364
patient controlled, 67, **274**
rib fractures, 8
anaphylaxis, 12–13, **144**
antepartum haemorrhage, 79,
80, **303**
anterior pituitary, hormones
secreted, 50, **236**
anticoagulants, **348**
direct oral, 95–96, **340–341**
antidepressants, 12, **142**
serotonin syndrome and, 55
antiemetics, 59, **258**
antiepileptics, **243**
antiparkinsonian drugs,
58, **257**
antiplatelet agents, 95–96,
340–341, 348
antithyroid drugs, **138**
antiviral drugs, **218**
aortic stenosis, 51
anaesthetic management, 51
ECG, 51, **239**
severity, **238**
Apfel score, 23, **171**
apnoea test, positive, 17
appendicectomy, 21
aprepitant, 23, **172**
aqueous humour, 25
Armitage 'rules', 7
arterial blood gas, 40
arterial ischaemia, **205**
arterio-venous (AV) fistula, 70
aspirin, 18, 95, 96, **340**
asthma, acute, 64–65, **268–269**
atlantoaxial instability, **186**
atrial fibrillation, 95, 98, 119
atropine, **362**
awake fibre-optic intubation
(AFOI), 34–35, **198–200**

back pain, chronic, 115
baclofen, 53, **244**
base of skull fracture, 85
benzodiazepines, **351**
bimaxillary osteotomy, 46–47,
228–229
bleomycin, 57, **253**
blood glucose levels, 40, 83,
210, 313
blood products, 118, **397**
blood transfusion, 117–118,
396–398
allogenic, 11
antepartum haemorrhage,
80, **304**
massive, 117, 118, **396**
blood viscosity, 36, **204**
body mass index (BMI), 46
Boerhaave syndrome, 45, **222**
Bolam test, **143**
bone cement implantation
syndrome (BCIS), 9–10,
135–136
bowel cancer, 116
brachial plexus, 93, **333–334**
approaches to, 93, **333**
bradycardia, 114
brain injury, traumatic, 84–85,
315–316
brainstem death, 16–17,
155–157
physiological derangements,
17, **156**
Bromage scale of motor
blockade, 104, **364**
bupivacaine, 69, **278, 361**
labour and, 103
placental transfer, 103
burn injuries, degrees of,
48, **233**

caesarean section
accidental awareness during,
32, **192**
local anaesthetic toxicity, 69
NICE guidelines on urgency,
7, **131**

placenta praevia and, 42, **215**
post-partum haemorrhage
  after, 66
cancer. *See also specific cancers*
hemicolectomy, 11
pain, 55, **247**
capnography, 59, **259**
capnometry, 59, **259**
carbamazepine, **162**
carbon dioxide measurement,
  59, **259–260**
carbon dioxide transport,
  120–121, **404–406**
carbon monoxide, **342**
carboprost, 67, **273**
carcinoid crisis, 83, **310**
carcinoid syndrome, 82–83,
  309–311
cardiac arrest. *See also heart
  headings*
  capnography role during,
  60, **260**
  local anaesthetic-induced, 70
cardiac bypass, 89–90, **324–325**
  off-pump, 112, **381–382**
cardiac implantable devices,
  100–101, **353–355**
cardiac output, 64, **266**
  monitoring, 108–109,
  374–376
cardiac resynchronisation
  device (CRT), 13, 14
  indications for, **147**
cardiac transplant, post, 15–16,
  152–154
cardiomyopathy
  dilated, 4–5, **125–126**
  post-partum, 115, **389**
  types of, 4, **125**
cardioplegia, 90, **324**
cardiopulmonary bypass
  circuit, 89
cardiopulmonary exercise
  testing, 73–74, 76, **289–290**
cardiothoracic surgery, 75
cardiotocography, 7
cardiovascular collapse, 9
cardiovascular physiology,
  managing, 4, **125**
Carlens double-lumen tube,
  76, **293**
carotid endarterectomy, 72–73,
  286–287
carotid stenosis, 72, **286**
cataracts, 98, **343–349**
caudal analgesia, 6, 7, **129–130**

caudal space, anatomy of, 6
cerebral hyperperfusion
  syndrome, **287**
cerebral palsy, 53, **243–244**
cerebrospinal fluid (CSF)
  flow, 3, **124**
  loss of, 245
cervical fixation, 15
cervical spinal cord injury, 26
cervical spinal fractures, 15
cervical spondylosis, **186**
chemotherapy, 56–57,
  252–254
child abuse, 17–18, **158–159**
Child–Pugh classes, 95, **339**
cholecystectomy, 71, 99
  laparoscopic, 15, 46
chronic allograft
  vasculopathy, 154
chronic liver disease, 94–95,
  337–339
chronic obstructive pulmonary
  disease (COPD), 8,
  76, 95
circle of Willis, 38
circumcision, 6, **129**
clinical flap observations, 37
coagulation cascade, 118
coagulation testing, 109–110,
  377–378
coagulopathy, **156**, **397**
Cobb angle, **322**
coeliac plexus, 54–55, **247–248**
colorectal surgery, 96
community-acquired
  pneumonia, 5
congenital heart disease, 39–40,
  208–209
consciousness, decreased, 62
corneal abrasions, 118, **399**
coronary artery disease, 112
corticosteroids, 21, **165**
cortisol, 117, **392**
cranial nerve palsy, 62, **263**
craniopharyngioma, 3
cricothyroidotomy, **242**
critical care airway, 52–53,
  241–242
critical care management
  pulmonary hypertension,
  78, **297**
critical illness myopathy, 127
cryoprecipitate, 118, **397**
CT scan
  carcinoid syndrome, 82
  meningitis, **330**

cuff-leak test, **200**
cycle ergometer, 73
cytokines, 116, **392**

dabigatran, 95–96, **340**
dapagliflozin, 83, **312**
day case surgery
  benefits of, 98, **347**
  child, 114, **386**
  diabetes and, 83–84, **312–314**
death, UK definition of, 16
deep hypothermic circulatory
  arrest, **325**
deep inferior epigastric
  perforator, 36
dehydration, severe, 41, 42, **212**
delirium, post-operative, **202**
dementia
  causes of, 35, **202**
  Parkinson's disease and, **257**
dental abscess, 34
dental injury, 119, **399**
dependence, 107, **372**
depression, ECT, 11, **142–143**
deprivation of liberties, 35–36,
  202–203
dexamethasone, 23, 84, 114,
  171, **385**
diabetes day case, 83–84,
  312–314
diabetic ketoacidosis (DKA),
  40–41, **210–211**
diamorphine, 104, **364**
diastolic dysfunction, **125**
diathermy, 100
difficult airway
  definition, 34, **198**
  Down's syndrome, 29
  Mallampati score, 60
  rheumatoid arthritis, 20
Difficult Airway Society
  guidelines, 35, **200**
dilated cardiomyopathy, 4–5,
  125–126
direct oral anticoagulants,
  95–96, **340–341**
discogenic pain, **191**
disseminated intravascular
  coagulation (DIC), 79, **303**
Doppler effect, 108, **374**
double-lumen tubes, 76, 77,
  223, **293**
Down's syndrome, 29,
  185–186
doxazocin, **196**
droperidol, 23, **171**

drug users, 22, **169**
dural sac, 6, **129**

echocardiography, 97, 108
  aortic stenosis, 51, **239**
  fractured neck of femur,
    120, **401**
  myotonic dystrophy, 99
EEG, depth of anaesthesia,
  32, **193**
electrocardiography (ECG)
  DKA, 41, **211**
  monitoring, **125**
  pacing activity, **353**
  pregnancy, 115
  right ventricular
    hypertrophy, 78, **297**
electroconvulsive therapy
  (ECT), 11, **142–143**
  electrode positioning,
    12, **142**
endocarditis, infective, 52, **239**
endocrine complications,
  pituitary disease, **236**
endometriosis, 23
endovascular aneurysm
  repair, 13
end-stage renal failure, 70, **280**
enhanced recovery, 116–117,
  392–394
enoximone, 28
enteral nutrition, 101
epidural block
  hernia surgery, 5
  labour, 103, **363**
  rib fractures, **133**
epidural space, 103, **363**
epigastric pain, 101
epilepsy, **379**
ergometrine, 67, 115, **273, 389**
esmolol, 112, **382**
evidence, levels of, 61, **262**
explicit awareness, **192**
external ventricular drain, 3
extra-articular disease, 20, **164**
extracorporeal membrane
  oxygenation (ECMO),
  113, **383**
eye injury, penetrating, 24–25,
  176–177
eye, anatomy, 24, **176**

facial trauma, 94, **335–336**
fascia iliaca block, 80–81,
  305–306
fat embolus, 105–106, **367–369**

femoral endarterectomy, 63
femoral fracture, 105
femur, fractured neck of,
  119–120, **401–403**
fentanyl, 103, **281**
ferromagnetic objects, 48, **231**
FEV 1, 76, **293**
fibreoptic intubation, awake,
  34–35, **198–200**
fluoxetine, 12, **142**
focal seizure, **379**
foetal blood samples, 7, **131**
foetal heart rate, 7, **131**
foetal well-being, 7, **131–132**
foreign body aspiration, 65–66,
  270–272
Forest plot, 60, **261**
fractured neck of femur,
  119–120, **401–403**
Frank–Starling
  mechanism, **265**
free flap surgery, 36–37,
  204–205
fresh frozen plasma, 118, **397**

gallstone disease, 15
gas induction, 66, **271**
general anaesthesia
  accidental awareness under,
    32, **192–193**
  depth of, 32
  nerve injuries and, 119, **399**
germ cell ovarian cancer, 56
gestational hypertension,
  18–19, **160–161**
Glasgow Coma Score, 38,
  84, **315**
gliclazide, 83, **312**
glyceryl trinitrate, 27, **181**
glycine, 105, **365**
glycopyrrolate, 103, 114,
  362, 385
glycosuria, 40, **210**
goal-directed fluid therapy, 117
GPAS guidelines, obstetric
  care, 92, **332**
Graves' disease, **138**
growth hormone, 117, **392**
Guillain–Barré syndrome,
  90–91, **326–327**
Gurd's minor criteria, 105, **367**

haematoma, post-
  thyroidectomy, 85–86,
  317–318
haemoglobin, 120, **404**

haemorrhage
  antepartum, 79, 80, **303**
  major, 117, **396**
  pelvic, **316**
  post-partum, 66–67, **273**
  post-tonsillectomy, 78–79,
    299–302
  subarachnoid, 38–39,
    206–207
haemorrhagic shock, **255**
Haldane effect, 121, **406**
HbA1c value, 83, **312**
heart disease. *See also cardiac
  headings*, ischaemic heart
  disease
  carcinoid syndrome and,
    82, **309**
  congenital, 39–40, **208–209**
heart failure, 63–64, **265–267**
  common causes of, 63, **265**
  mechanism types, **265**
heart murmur, 114, 120, **385**
HELLP, **160**
hemicolectomy,
  laparoscopic, 11
heparin, 90, **324**
hepatic encephalopathy, **337**
hepatitis B, 22, **169**
hepatitis C, 22, **169**
hernia repair, cardiomyopathy
  and, 4–5
high-flow nasal oxygen
  therapy, 32, **194**
hip fracture, 80, **305**
hip replacement, 9–10,
  135–136
hip surgery, 119, 120, **401**
HIV, 22
  caesarean section and, **132**
hormones, anterior pituitary,
  50, **236**
HPV infection, **194**
hydrocephalus, 3, **123–124**
  signs and symptoms, **123**
hypercalcaemia, 44, **220**
hypercapnoea, 17, **157**
hyperglycaemia, 40, **210**
hypersensitivity, anaphylaxis
  and, 13, **144**
hypertension, 71–72, **283–284**
  BCIS and, 9
  gestational, 18–19, **160–161**
  phaeochromocytoma and, 33
  pulmonary, 77–78, **296–298**
hyperthermia, malignant,
  21–22, **167–168**

hyperthyroidism, 10, **137–139**
  signs and symptoms, **137**
hypertrophic cardiomyopathy, 4, **125**
hypocalcaemia, 44, **220**
hypoglycaemic agents, 83, **312**
hypo-osmolality, **366**
hypotension, 117
  anaphylaxis and, **144**
  BCIS and, **135**
  carcinoid syndrome, 83
  ischaemic heart disease, 28
hypothermia
  cardiac bypass and, 90, **325**
  neonates and, 102, **360**
hypoxaemia, 76
hypoxia, 9, 121, **209**, **405**
hysterectomy, 94

ibuprofen, 67, 114, **385**
ICU acquired weakness (ICUAW), 5–6, **127–128**
idarucizumab, **341**
immunoglobin-G (IgG), 291
immunoglobulin therapy, 90, **327**
immunology, anaphylaxis and, 13, **144**
immunosuppression, 16, **153**
implantable cardioverter defibrillator (ICD), 100, 355
implicit awareness, **192**
Independent Mental Capacity Advocate (IMCA), **203**
infra-red spectroscopy, 59, **259**
inhaled foreign body, 65–66, **270–272**
insulin-like growth factor 1 (IGF-1), 50, **235**
interscalene block, 93, **333**
intra-abdominal pressure, raised, 46
intracranial haemorrhage, 96
intracranial pressure (ICP), rise in, 3, **124**
Intralipid, 70
intraocular pressure, 25
intravenous resuscitation fluid, 49
iron therapy, 393
irrigation fluid, 105, **365**
ischaemic heart disease, 27–28, 108, **181–182**, **205**, **280**
Ivor Lewis oesophagectomy, 73

ketonaemia, 40, **210**
King's College criteria, **308**
knee arthroscopy, 83
knee replacement, 20, 95

labetalol, 18, 19
labour analgesia, 103–104, **363–364**
landmark technique, 73, 80
laparoscopy
  adrenalectomy, 33
  anterior resection, 116
  cholecystectomy, 15, 46, 71, 99
  endometriosis, 23
  hemicolectomy, 11
  obesity and, 46, **225–227**
  sigmoidectomy, 58
laparotomy, 108, 115
  emergency, 117
  perforated diverticulum, 27
laryngeal mask airway, 48
laryngoscopy, 25
larynx, muscles of the, 34, **199**
laser, 121–122, **407–409**
lateral positioning, 45
Le Fort fractures, 94, **335**
Lee's revised cardiac index, 27
left ventricular end-diastolic pressure (LVEDP), 63, **265**
left ventricular hypertrophy, 51
left ventricular pressure-volume loop, 63, **265**
lidocaine, **271**
lignocaine, 35, 69, **278**, **361**, **391**
lipid emulsion, 70
liver disease, 94–95, **337–339**
liver transplant, 82, **308**
lobectomy, 76
local anaesthesia. *See* regional anaesthesia
low back pain, 30–32, **190–191**
  psychosocial factors, 31, **191**
lumbar facet joint pain, **191**
lung adenocarcinoma, 76

MACOCHA score, 52, **241**
magnesium, **161**
magnesium sulphate, **197**
magnetic resonance imaging (MRI), 47–48, **230–232**
  labour, 104, **364**
  trigeminal neuralgia, 19
major haemorrhage, 117, **396**

malignant hyperthermia, 21–22, **167–168**
Mallampati score, 60
massive transfusion, 117, 118, **396**
maternal collapse in labour, 30, **188**
maximal oxygen consumption, **293**
mean arterial pressure, 108, **374**
meningitis, 91–92, **329–330**
Mental Capacity Act 2005, 35
mental capacity, liberties and, 35–36, **202–203**
meta-analysis, 60, **261**
Metabolic Equivalent of a Task (MET), 73, **289**
metformin, 83, **312**
metoclopramide, 23
morphine, 67, 116, **133**, **391**
  liver disease and, 95, **338**
motor evoked potentials (MEPs), **149**, **323**
motor neuron action potential, 21
multiple endocrine neoplasia, **221**
Murray score, 113, **383**
muscle contraction, 21
muscle relaxants, **149**
muscle spasms, 53, **244**
myasthenia gravis, 75–76, **291–292**
myasthenic crisis, 75, **292**
mycophenolate, **153**
mycophenolate mofetil, 16
myocardial oxygen supply and demand, 27, **181**
myotomes, upper limb, 26
myotonic dystrophy, 99–100, **350–352**

N-acetyl cysteine (NAC), 81, **146**, **307**
National Audit Project (NAP) 4, 52
nausea, post-operative, 23, **171–172**
nebulisers, **268**
necrosectomy, **357**
needlestick injury, 22, **169**
Neisseria meningitidis, 92
neo-adjuvant chemotherapy, 56, 57, **252**

neostigmine, 103, **362**
neprilysin, **266**
nerve injuries, 119, **399**
neuroleptic malignant
    syndrome, **249**
neuromuscular blockade, **143**
neuropathic pain, **247**
neurotoxicity, 57, **254**
Newtonian fluid, laminar flow,
    36, **204**
NICE guidelines
    caesarean section, 7, **131**
    hip fracture analgesia,
        80, **305**
nicotine, 96, **342**
nitrous oxide, 106–107,
    370–371
nocturnal dyspnoea, 64
noradrenaline, **196**
norepinephrine, **310**
not for cardiopulmonary
    resuscitation decision, 36
NSAIDs, **133**
    avoidance of, **281**

obesity
    categories of, 46, **225**
    laparoscopy and, 46,
        225–227
obstructive sleep apnoea (OSA)
    Down's syndrome and, **186**
    obesity and, 46, **225**
octreotide, 82, 83, **310**
odansetron, 171
oesophageal Doppler, 108,
    117, **375**
oesophageal rupture, 45,
    222–224
off-pump cardiac bypass, 112,
    381–382
ondansetron, 23, 114, **385**
one-lung ventilation, 76–77,
    293–294
opioids, **385**, *See also* morphine
    abuse of, **372**
    withdrawal, 116
oral glucose tolerance test
    (OGTT), 50
organ donation, 16–17,
    155–157
oropharyngeal cancer,
    32, **194**
oxycodone, 115, 116, **391**
oxygen binding, 121, **404**
oxygen debt, 74, **290**
oxygen pulse, **290**

oxygen transport, 120–121,
    404–406
oxytocin, 115, **389**

pacemaker code, 100, **353**
packed red blood cells, 118
paediatric drug doses, 114
pain
    assessment in children,
        7, **130**
    cancer, 55, **247**
    epigastric, 101
    labour and, 103, **363**
    low back, 30–32, **190–191**
    phantom limb, 67–68,
        274–275
    post-herpetic neuralgia, **218**
pancreatic cancer, 54
pancreatitis, 101, **356–357**
panendoscopy, 32
papilloedema, **123**
paracetamol, 67, 71, 114, **385**
    overdose, 81–82, **307–308**
parathyroid adenoma, 44
parathyroid glands, 44, **219**
parathyroid hormone (PTH),
    44, **220**
parathyroidectomy, 44–45,
    219–221
paravertebral block, **133**
Parkinson's disease, 58–59,
    257–258
    classic triad, 58, **257**
Parkland formula, **233**
patient-controlled analgesia
    (PCA), 67, **274**
peak velocity, **375**
pelvic injury, traumatic, 84–85,
    315–316
percutaneous endoscopic
    gastrostomy, 53
permanent pacemaker,
    100, **354**
peroneal nerve palsy, 119, **399**
petechial rash, **367**
phaeochromocytoma, 33–34,
    196–197
phantom limb pain, 67–68,
    274–275
pharmacokinetic models,
    24, **174**
phenelzine, 12, **142**
phenoxybenzamine, **196**
phrenic nerve palsy, **333**
physical injuries, **118–119**,
    399–400

pituitary disease, 50–51,
    235–237
placenta, 102–103, **361–362**
    abnormal adherence, 43
    drug transfer across,
        102, **361**
placenta praevia, 42–43,
    215–216
    grades of, 42, **215**
placental abruption, 79–80,
    303–304
plasmapheresis, **327**
platelets, 118, **397**
pneumonia
    acute severe, 113
    community-acquired, 5
pneumoperitoneum, 46
point-of-care coagulation
    testing, 109–110, **377–378**
    trace abnormalities, 109, **378**
polyuria, 219
population inversion, 121, **407**
positive end expiratory
    pressure (PEEP), 77,
        195, 294
post-cardiac transplant, 15–16,
    152–154
post-dural puncture headache,
    54, **245–246**
posterior fossa tumours,
    62, **264**
post-herpetic neuralgia, 43–44,
    217–218
post-operative nausea and
    vomiting, 23, **171–172**
    drugs used, 23, **171**
post-partum cardiomyopathy,
    115, **388**
post-partum haemorrhage,
    66–67, **273**
    pharmacological
        management, 66, **273**
post-thyroidectomy
    haematoma, 85–86,
        317–318
post-tonsillectomy
    haemorrhage, 78–79,
        299–302
prasugrel, 95, 96, **340**
prednisolone, 20, **165**
pre-eclampsia, 18–19, **160–161**
    common symptoms, 18
pregabalin, 115
preload, 108, **374**
pre-operative anaemia, 11,
    140–141, 393

prilocaine, 69, **278**
primary hypertension, 71, **283**
primary postpartum
    haemorrhage, 66, **273**
primary post-tonsillectomy
    haemorrhage, 78, **299**
prone position, 15, **149–151**
propofol, 24
propofol-related infusion
    syndrome, 28–29, **183–184**
    mortality from, **183**
proteinuria, 19, **160**
psoas compartment block,
    120, **402**
psychosocial factors, low back
    pain, 31, **191**
puerperal sepsis, 92–93,
    331–332
pulmonary artery pressure, 78,
    294, 296
pulmonary hypertension,
    77–78, **296–298**
    WHO categories, 77, **296**
pulmonary toxicity, 57, **253**
pulmonary vascular
    resistance, **209**
pyloric stenosis, 41–42,
    212–214
pyloromyotomy, 42

ramipril, 4
Ranson's criteria, **357**
rapid sequence induction, 25
red blood cell (RBC) sickling,
    68, **276**
red blood cells, 118, **397**
regional anaesthesia
    carotid endarterectomy,
        72, **286**
    cataracts, 98, **348**
    circumcision, **129**
    diabetes and, 84, **313**
    enhanced recovery and, **394**
    rib fractures, 8
    spinal cord stimulator
        and, 116
    techniques, **133**
regional anaesthetics
    maximum doses, 69, **278**
    toxicity, 69–70, **278–279**
relapse, 107, **373**
remifentanil, 149, **264**
renal transplant, 70–71,
    280–281
restricted cardiomyopathy,
    4, **125**

resuscitation
    cardiopulmonary, 70, **279**
    management, 57, **255**
    post-tonsillectomy
        haemorrhage, 79, **300**
rheumatoid arthritis, 20–21,
    93, **164–166, 334**
    extra-articular disease,
        20, **164**
rib fixation, **134**
rib fractures, **133–134**
    analgesia, 8
    pulmonary complications
        and, 8, **133**
    regional anaesthesia, 8
right ventricular hypertrophy,
    78, **297**
rivaroxaban, 95, 96, **340**
Robertshaw double-lumen
    tube, 76, **293**
rocuronium, 95, **338**
ropivacaine, 69, **278, 361**

sacroiliac joint pain, **191**
schizophrenia, 84
scoliosis, 88–89, **322–323**
secondary hypertension,
    71, **283**
secondary postpartum
    haemorrhage, 67
secondary post-tonsillectomy
    haemorrhage, 78, **299**
seizure, 111, **379–380**
sensitivity, clinical test, 60, **261**
serotonin receptor subtypes,
    56, **251**
serotonin syndrome, 55–56,
    249–251
serratus plane block, **134**
severe acute pancreatitis, 101
Severinghaus electrode, 60, **260**
sevoflurane, 66
shingles, 43, **217**
shoulder replacement, 93
sialhorrhoea, **257**
sick sinus syndrome, 100
sickle cell disease, 68–69,
    276–277
sigmoid carcinoma, 35
sigmoidectomy, 58
sildenafil, **297**
smoking, 96–97, **342**
somatic pain, 103, **247, 363**
somatosensory evoked
    potentials (SSEPs),
    149, 323

sore throat, post-operative,
    119, **400**
specialist burns centre,
    49, **234**
specificity, clinical test, 60, **261**
spinal anaesthesia, 54, 96,
    115, **245**
    TURP, 104
spinal cord injury, 26–27, 88,
    178–179
spinal cord monitoring, 15
spinal cord stimulator,
    115–116, **390–391**
spleen, functions of, 57, **256**
splenectomy, 57–58, **255–256**
spontaneous emission,
    121, **407**
statistics, 60–61, **261–262**
Sternbach criteria, 55, **249**
stimulated emission, 121, **407**
stop before you block
    process, 80
STOP-BANG
    questionnaire, 46
strabismus surgery, 114,
    385–386
Streptococcus, **331**
stroke volume, 63, 97, **265**
stump pain, **274**
subarachnoid haemorrhage,
    38–39, **206–207**
substance abuse, 107–108,
    372–373
    risk factors, 107, **372**
sub-Tenon's block, 98, **348**
suicide attempt, 81
superconductivity, 48, **231**
superficial cervical plexus
    block, 73, **287**
surgical stress response,
    116, **392**
Swan–Ganz catheter, **374**
sympathetic lysis, 55
syntocinon, 67, **273**
systemic vascular resistance
    (SVR), **126, 153, 209, 239**
systolic dysfunction, **125**

tachycardia, 112, 117
tacrolimus, 16, **153**
tadalafil, **297**
target controlled infusion
    (TCI) pump, 24
tetralogy of Fallot, 39, **209**
thiopental, 95, **338**
thoracic epidurals, 82

three-compartment model, pharmacokinetics, 24, **174**
throat pack, retained, 47, **229**
thromboelastography, 110, **378**
thyroid function tests, 10
thyroid hormones, 10, **137**
thyroidectomy, 10, **138**
  post-haematoma, 85–86, **317–318**
tobacco, **194**
tolerance, 107, **372**
tonic–clonic seizure, 19, 111
tonsillar hypertrophy, 32
tonsillectomy, post-haemorrhage, 78–79, **299–302**
total intravenous anaesthesia, 23–24, 47, **173–174**
toxicity, local anaesthetic, 69–70, **278–279**
tracheoesophageal fistula, 101–102, **358–360**
tracheostomy, critical care patients, 52
tranexamic acid, 118, **315**
transient ischaemic attack, 72, **286**

transplants
  liver, 82, **308**
  post-cardiac, 15–16, **152–154**
  renal, 70–71, **280–281**
trans-tracheal block, 35
transurethral resection of prostate, 104
transurethral resection syndrome, 104–105, **365–366**
trauma, 57–58, **255–256**
  lethal triad of, 118, **396**
traumatic pelvic and brain injury, 84–85, **315–316**
trigeminal neuralgia, 19–20, **162–163**
  surgical options, 20, **163**
trisomy 21, **185**
tubeless surgery, 32–33, **194–195**

UK Obstetric Surveillance criteria, 30, **188**
ultrasound, 97–98, **342–343**
  interscalene block, 93, **333**
  principles of, **344**
upper limb myotomes, 26
uterine cancer, 94

vaccinations, bacterial, 58, **256**
vagus nerve, 86–87, **320–321**
Valsalva manoeuvre, 86, **318**
valvular heart disease, 51–52, **237–239**
varicella zoster virus (VZV), **217**
vasopressors, 83, **310**
venous blood gas, 41
ventilator settings, 65, **269**
ventriculoperitoneal (VP) shunt, blocked, 3
verapamil, 112, **382**
vertebra, anatomy, 31, **190**
vincristine, **254**
visceral pain, 103, **363**
vocal cord polypectomy, 121
vomiting, post-operative, 23, **171–172**

warfarin, 95, 96, 98, 119, 120, **340, 348, 403**
White double-lumen tube, 76, **293**

zero-order kinetics, 24, **174**

Printed in the United States
by Baker & Taylor Publisher Services